Contents

First Printing

Bottom Line Books® publishes the advice of expert authorities in many fields. These opinions may
at times conflict as there are often different approaches to solving problems. The use of this
material is no substitute for health, legal, accounting or other professional services.
Consult competent professionals for answers to your specific questions.

Telephone numbers, addresses, prices, offers and Web sites listed in this book are accurate
at the time of publication, but they are subject to frequent change.

Bottom Line Books® is a registered trademark of
Boardroom® Inc.
281 Tresser Boulevard, Stamford, CT 06901

www.bottomlinepublications.com

Printed in the United States of America

BLHL/am

SPECIAL REPORT #1:

Healing Secrets Doctors Don't Tell You

Healing Secrets Doctors Don't Tell You

Preventing Illness with Fish or Fish Oil

When talk turns to foods that contribute to longevity, fish is inevitably mentioned—along with fruits, vegetables and whole grains.

In clinical trials involving patients with life-threatening ailments, patients who regularly eat fish live longer than similar patients who don't eat fish or who eat it only occasionally.

But not all fish is the same. For maximum benefit, you must choose the right *kind* of fish.

OMEGA-3 FATTY ACIDS

We've known for decades that eating fish helps prevent illness and death, but only within the last 20 years have we been able to pinpoint the specific disease-fighting agent in fish.

The active agent is actually a pair of polyunsaturated fats. These *omega-3* fatty acids—*eicosapentaenoic acid* (EPA) and *docosahexaenoic acid* (DHA)—help lower triglycerides. EPA is converted into prostaglandins which have anti-inflammatory activity. The level of triglycerides tends to rise after meals, thereby raising the risk for heart attack.

In addition, omega-3s are known to help prevent arrhythmias.

Omega-3s have also been shown in laboratory studies to inhibit tumor growth…and to keep cancer cells from spreading.

GETTING THE MOST FROM FISH

Some researchers report that just one meal of fish per week confers significant protection against heart attack. But recent evidence suggests that to maximize the overall health benefits of eating fish, you must eat it two or three times per week. Eating fish more frequently does not seem to confer any additional protection.

Key: Choosing fish whose flesh is rich in omega-3 fatty acids. In general, fatty fish that live in deep, cold water have high levels of omega-3s.

Artemis P. Simopoulos, MD, president of the Center for Genetics, Nutrition and Health in Washington, DC. She is also coauthor of *The Omega Plan: The Medically Proven Diet That Restores Your Body's Essential Nutritional Balance.* HarperCollins.

The chart below lists the total content of EPA plus DHA, in grams (g) per half-cup serving...

mackerel	2.5 g	lake whitefish	1.3 g
herring	1.7 g	tuna	1.3 g
lake trout	1.6 g	Atlantic salmon	1.2 g
chinook salmon	1.4 g	bluefish	1.2 g

Don't worry that eating fish will cause you to "overdose" on fat. Even the fattiest fish are relatively lean. Ounce for ounce, they contain about as much fat as the leanest cuts of beef.

Best ways to cook fish: Poaching, baking, broiling or grilling. Corn oil and other oils typically used for frying or sautéing are rich in omega-6 fatty acids, which tend to neutralize omega-3s.

SAFETY CONCERNS

Fish oil does slow blood-clotting, but this has never been shown to cause uncontrolled bleeding or any other health problem—even among people who undergo surgery. It's recommended to discontinue use one week before surgery.

In some studies, people have suffered no ill effects even after taking up to 5 g of EPA plus DHA a day for seven years. Still, it's prudent to discuss fish oil supplementation with a doctor if you...

...have asthma. Some asthmatics report an increased frequency of asthma attacks when they take fish oil capsules.

...have diabetes. Dosages higher than 3 g a day can cause elevated blood glucose levels.

...are taking an anticoagulant, such as *heparin* or *warfarin* (Coumadin).

Let Oregano Help Keep You Healthy

Ounce for ounce, oregano has 42 times more antioxidant activity than apples... 30 times more than potatoes...and 12 times more than oranges. One tablespoon of fresh oregano (or one-half teaspoon dried oregano) contains the same amount of antioxidants as one medium-sized apple.

Other antioxidant-packed herbs are chives, coriander, dill, parsley, sage and thyme.

Helpful: Add herbs to hot water for a potent tea...or sprinkle them on lean meats and vegetables.

Shiow Y. Wang, PhD, a plant physiologist and biochemist, US Department of Agriculture, Beltsville, MD. Her study was published in the *Journal of Agricultural and Food Chemistry.*

Cooked Carrots Are More Nutritious Than Raw

Antioxidant levels increased more than 34% after carrots were cooked—and continued to increase while the vegetables were kept at 104°F for one week. Heating softens the carrot tissue, triggering the release of antioxidants attached to cell walls. This phenomenon may also occur in other vegetables.

Luke Howard, PhD, professor of food science, University of Arkansas, Fayetteville. Dr. Howard's research was published in the *Journal of Agricultural and Food Chemistry.*

Eat More Prunes to Prevent Bone Loss

In one finding, 58 postmenopausal women who consumed about 12 prunes per day for three months showed higher blood levels of enzymes and growth factors indicative of bone formation than women who did not eat prunes.

Theory: The polyphenolic compounds and other nutrients in prunes act as antioxidants to curb bone loss. Although women were studied, researchers believe that men can gain the same beneficial effects from eating prunes.

Bonus: Those studied suffered no significant gastrointestinal side effects.

Bahram H. Arjmandi, PhD, RD, chair and Margaret A. Sitton Professor, Dept. of Nutrition, Food & Exercise Sciences, Florida State University, Tallahassee.

Rev Up Your Immunity With Nature's Remedies

Robert Rountree, MD, family practitioner specializing in nutrition, herbology and mind/body therapy, located in Boulder, CO. He is also a member of the American Herbalists Guild and is coauthor of *Immunotics: A Revolutionary Way to Fight Infection, Beat Chronic Illness and Stay Well.* Perigee.

We live our lives in a veritable soup of viruses, bacteria, fungi and other disease-causing agents.

The immune system—which consists of billions of specialized cells located throughout the body—is on the lookout for these disease-causing invaders. But it doesn't always work as well as we'd like.

Do you seem to catch all of the "bugs" that come along? Your immune system might be sabotaged by chronic psychological stress… environmental toxins, like mercury, arsenic or dioxin…and/or poor nutritional choices.

Immunity-zapping foods: Alcohol, margarine, commercially baked goods and other sources of hydrogenated and partially hydrogenated fat, sugary foods and hot dogs, bacon and other cured meats that contain cancer-causing food additives.

Unfortunately, immune system problems that lead to frequent minor illness can also raise the risk for certain forms of cancer.

Good news: It's possible to boost a flagging immune system or fortify a healthy one with immunity-boosting foods, herbs, supplements and lifestyle changes.

NATURAL IMMUNITY BOOSTERS*

•**Aloe vera.** Two ounces of the juice of this succulent, subtropical plant every two hours for up to 12 hours works as an anti-inflammatory to help relieve diarrhea, colitis or irritable bowel syndrome. As an alternative, you can take one-half to two teaspoons of freeze-dried aloe vera dissolved in water or juice daily. Applied topically, aloe vera gel speeds healing of sunburn, minor wounds and burns.

*Immunity-boosting products can be purchased in health-food stores.

•**Astragalus.** This herb helps curb chronic colds, ear infections and the flu. It also helps restore immunity in cancer patients who have been affected by chemotherapy drugs.

Typical dosage: One 500-milligram (mg) capsule—or about 15 drops of tincture daily.

•**Berries.** Blackberries, blueberries, cranberries and strawberries contain immunity-boosting *anthocyanidins* and other flavonoids. They also contain lots of dietary fiber and vitamin C—both known cancer fighters.

•**Carrots, sweet potatoes, tomatoes and yellow squash.** Brightly colored vegetables contain *carotenoids,* compounds known to prevent cancers of the lung, colon, breast, uterus and prostate.

•**Cruciferous vegetables.** Broccoli, brussels sprouts, cabbage, cauliflower, collard greens and kale protect against breast, cervical and other cancers, according to research conducted at Rockefeller University in New York City and Johns Hopkins University School of Medicine in Baltimore.

•**Garlic, onions, chives and leeks** are loaded with sulfur compounds, which have potent antimicrobial and antifungal properties. These "allium" vegetables are effective against colds, flu, parasites, yeast overgrowth and stomach "bugs." Garlic may even help prevent and treat prostate cancer, according to research conducted at Memorial Sloan-Kettering Cancer Center in New York City.

Typical dosage: One or two cloves of raw garlic a day. If you dislike garlic odor, take one to three capsules of freeze-dried garlic daily.

Reputable brands: Enzymatic Therapy's Garlinase and Nature's Way Garlicin.

•**Grapefruit seed extract.** In addition to the standard food-safety precautions, take 15 drops daily in a glass of juice upon arrival in an underdeveloped location to help prevent traveler's diarrhea.

Important: Ask your doctor before taking grapefruit seed extract. It may interfere with some medications.

•**Green tea.** It contains *polyphenols,* antioxidant compounds that stop formation of *nitrosamines,* cancer-causing compounds produced in the stomach.

Green tea drinkers have low rates of pancreatic, esophageal, colon, stomach and lung cancers. Drink three to four cups or take two to four 500-mg capsules of green tea extract daily.

•**Nutritional supplements.** In addition to vitamin C, you may want to take other natural immunity boosters daily. *Some to consider…*

   •Carotenoids (10,000 international units—IU)

   •Coenzyme Q10 (50 mg)

   •Lipoic acid (50 mg)

   •Selenium (100 micrograms—mcg)

   •Vitamin E (200 IU)

   •Zinc (20 mg)

•**Soy foods.** Tofu, soy milk, tempeh and miso contain antioxidants and phytochemicals that help block tumor growth. Tofu, specifically, is believed to reduce the risk for prostate cancer.

EVERYDAY HABITS

To stay healthy, incorporate these simple strategies into your daily life…

•**Clean cutting boards thoroughly.** Use a diluted bleach solution and air-dry. Do so each time the board comes into contact with meat, poultry or fish. Buy wood boards—they are easier to clean than plastic. And always use separate boards for meats and other foods.

•**Get plenty of sleep.** Lack of sleep—even for a single night—dramatically reduces the activity of a key immune system component known as *natural killer cells.*

•**Keep your windows open.** An overheated, stuffy room is the perfect breeding ground for germs that cause colds and flu.

•**Wash your hands often.** Do so before eating or preparing food and after going to the bathroom. Wash more often when you're around sick people.

IMMUNITY AND ATTITUDE

Even when following a healthful diet and lifestyle, you will get sick occasionally. But optimism can help you get well.

Just as positive emotions help boost immunity, negative ones reduce immunity. They do so by triggering secretion of the stress hormone *cortisol,* which inhibits the inflammatory response and raises blood pressure.

When you're faced with a health crisis, help your immune system by working to overcome negative thoughts. Join a support group and/or get psychotherapy.

Caution: Never rely on your mind as the sole treatment for serious illness. Always seek appropriate medical therapy.

WHAT ABOUT ANTIBIOTICS?

When antibiotics came into use more than 50 years ago, it seemed they could zap any bacteria—even those that cause tuberculosis and meningitis.

Unfortunately, the decades of overuse have rendered these drugs ineffective against certain "bugs." And, of course, we now know that antibiotics wipe out beneficial bacteria along with the disease-causing ones.

Bottom line: Use the immunity-boosters to stay healthy and to speed recovery from illnesses you would normally treat without calling your doctor—colds, mild sore throats and stomach ailments.

Caution: If you're experiencing high fever, vomiting, chest pain or dizziness, you may need a course of antibiotics or some other treatment. Call your doctor.

Intestinal Bacteria for Better Digestion, Stronger Immunity and Disease Prevention

Elizabeth Lipski, PhD, CCN, in private practice in Asheville, NC. She is the author of Digestive Wellness. McGraw-Hill. For more about beneficial bacteria, visit www.innova tivehealing.com.

The human intestinal tract is home for more than 100 trillion bacteria. Two species of digestive bacteria, in particular—*Lactobacillus acidophilus* (*L. acidophilus*) and *Bifidobacterium* (*bifidus* or *bifidum*)—help protect our health in significant ways.

•**They limit growth of the fungus *Candida albicans*** and other harmful microbes. Candida can cause many health problems, including eye, nail, vaginal and throat infections.

•**They prevent food poisoning** by producing natural antibiotics to control *salmonella* and other pathogens…and by increasing immune function in the intestines.

•**They synthesize vitamins A and K.** Vitamin A helps to maintain good vision and healthy skin. Vitamin K assists blood clotting and bone formation.

•**They synthesize B vitamins,** which help to fight psychological and physical stress. The bacteria also generate acids that help facilitate absorption of minerals…and break down protein into amino acids. The body uses these acids to manufacture and repair hormones and enzymes and maintain bone structure.

•**They facilitate digestion** by breaking down lactose in dairy products, creating lactic acid that helps acidify the digestive tract to prevent overgrowth of harmful bacteria. They also help regulate bowel movements and help prevent traveler's diarrhea.

•**They help prevent cancer** by limiting the growth of bacteria that produce cancer-causing *nitrates*. Bacteria also metabolize and eliminate carcinogens, such as pesticides.

BOOSTING GOOD BACTERIA

It's important to make sure good bacteria reproduce faster than they die…

•**Load up on fruits and vegetables.** They create a healthy intestinal environment. Eat at least nine half-cup servings every day.

•**Eat fermented foods.** These contain bacteria —often the beneficial kind. Eat them at least four times a week.

Examples: Yogurt, sauerkraut, tofu, miso (a soy-based condiment), tamari (a type of soy sauce), tempeh (soybean cake) and pickles.

Preservatives like *sodium benzoate* destroy friendly bacteria in pickles and fermented foods. Choose brands that are preservative-free.

•**Go easy on sugar and alcohol.** Disease-causing bacteria and fungi feed on sugar—especially the refined variety in table sugar, sweets and alcohol.

•**Avoid or limit consumption of refined flour products,** such as white bread and pasta.

•**Drink green tea.** It contains *polyphenols*—natural compounds that maintain a balance of beneficial bacteria in the gastrointestinal tract.

Bonus: Catechins in green tea help fight off cancer, control blood sugar and strengthen bones. Drink four cups a day.

•**Try ginseng.** This herb promotes growth of friendly bacteria. Ask your doctor about having two cups of ginseng tea or taking two ginseng capsules daily.

Caution: Some ginseng brands have been found to contain pesticides and lead. You can find contaminant-free brands at *www.consumer lab.com.*

PROBIOTIC SUPPLEMENTS

Another way to increase levels of friendly bacteria in your system is to take a supplement that contains *L. acidophilus* and/or *bifidus*. These are known as "probiotics."

Purchase freeze-dried capsules or powder. Liquid supplements tend to lose their potency quickly.

Buy only the refrigerated supplements, and promptly put them in the refrigerator when you bring them home.

Some of the high-quality brands include Natren, Essential Formulas, Jarrow and Ethical Nutrients. They are available in most health-food stores.

A typical supplement dosage for general health is one billion microbes each of *L. acidophilus* and *bifidus.*

Helpful: Take probiotic supplements on an empty stomach—and never with hot liquids. Heat kills bacteria.

At first, probiotics can cause a massive die-off of unfriendly bacteria. Although desirable, this can lead to bloating and gas.

Solution: Cut back to just a few pinches daily. Break open a capsule to get this amount. Increase the dose in small increments when the problem goes away—usually within days.

TREATING DISEASE

Probiotics can prevent or resolve *dysbiosis* —excess unfriendly bacteria in the digestive tract that can trigger or complicate a variety of health conditions, such as…

•**Diarrhea induced by antibiotics.** Antibiotics destroy bad *and* good bacteria. This can bring on diarrhea. Take up to 10 billion microbes of probiotics daily during a course of antibiotics—until the diarrhea goes away.

• **Vaginal infections.** *L. acidophilus* helps maintain and restore vaginal health. For acute infections, take one to two billion microbes of probiotics daily.

• **Candida.** One to two billion microbes daily helps counter this fungal infection. Take for several months.

• **Bad breath.** It is often caused by bacterial fermentation in the intestinal tract. One billion microbes of probiotics per day helps treat the problem.

• **Constipation.** Poor bowel health can lead to an inefficient digestive system. One billion microbes of probiotic powder every day helps restore regularity.

• **Lactose intolerance.** Although it's not a cure, one billion microbes of probiotics taken daily reduces gas and bloating. First—try dairy products with added *L. acidophilus*.

• **Diverticular disease.** Probiotics help fight infections from this painful condition, in which pea-sized pouches balloon out along the intestinal wall, primarily in the colon.

Take two billion microbes daily during a flare-up, or take one billion microbes daily for prevention.

• **Chronic fatigue.** One billion microbes of probiotics daily improves digestion, which is almost always compromised in people with this condition.

More from Dr. Elizabeth Lipski...

Bowel Transit Time Can Reveal a Lot About Your Health

Bowel transit time—how long it takes what you eat to move from your mouth and out of your body—reveals a lot about your health.

Helpful: Eat three beets or swallow 2 grams of activated charcoal (sold over-the-counter in drugstores and health-food stores). Note when you do this and when you see dark-red or black stool. That's your transit time. *Rules of thumb...*

• **More than 24 hours**—Stool is staying in your colon too long, perhaps allowing toxins to be reabsorbed into the bloodstream. Boost fiber intake...and drink at least eight eight-ounce glasses of water every day.

• **12 to 24 hours**—Your bowel function is normal.

• **Less than 12 hours**—This is too quick. Your body may not have enough time to absorb the nutrients it needs. See your doctor.

Helpful Acupressure Points

Acupressure can help relieve nausea, fatigue and more. Stimulate acupressure points once or twice daily. Use the thick, padded part of the thumbs to press firmly and evenly on these points.

• **For nausea**—Point C.

• **For fatigue and weakness**—Points B and C.

• **For abdominal cramping and diarrhea**—Points A and B.

• **For immune system regulation**—Point B.

Illustration by Shawn Banner.

Robert G. Gish, MD, associate clinical professor of medicine at the University of California San Francisco School of Medicine, and medical director of the liver transplant program at California Pacific Medical Center, *www.cpmc. org/liver.*

Cancer Survival Secrets

The late Richard Bloch, a philanthropist in Kansas City, MO, and cofounder of the tax-preparation firm H&R Block, Inc. In 1978, Bloch was diagnosed with terminal lung cancer and given three months to live. He survived for six more years.

Almost from the minute a diagnosis of cancer is confirmed, the advice begins pouring in—from your doctor...your parents...your spouse...your friends.

But perhaps no one is better equipped to tell you how to beat the disease than cancer survivors themselves. *Here are their strategies for making it through the difficult times...*

• **Get a second opinion as soon as possible after your initial diagnosis.** Ideally, you will obtain opinions from several specialists, including a medical oncologist, a radiation oncologist and a surgeon.

Richard Bloch, who survived lung cancer for over two decades, was such a believer in this approach that he founded a free, multidisciplinary second-opinion panel staffed by more than 100 physicians in his native Kansas City, Missouri.

"I believe that one out of every four patients the panel saw had his or her life saved because of the panel," Bloch said.

• **Commit yourself to doing everything in your power to beat the disease.** "This might sound silly," said Bloch, "but some people just turn everything over to their doctors and expect them to fix it."

You must become intimately involved in all aspects of your cancer treatment. It's tempting, of course, to leave the details to the doctors. But to maximize your chances of survival, you have to muster all of your resources and exhaust every option open to you.

• **Expect the first three months after the diagnosis to be awful.** That advice comes from Daniel Kohn, a therapist who was diagnosed with a brain tumor in 1997.

"You're going to be in shock and in denial, no matter how well-equipped you are," he said. "Just ride it through. It gets better."

• **Pick doctors who are affiliated with a major hospital.** Fight for your right to have the doctor you choose, no matter what your insurance company says.

• **Look beyond your family for emotional support.** When Bloch was diagnosed, the few cancer survivors he knew didn't seem interested in talking with him. So he launched a cancer hotline (800-433-0464 or *www.blochcancer.org*), which utilizes a volunteer group of cancer patients who take phone calls from newly diagnosed cancer patients.

Many cancer patients find support groups especially helpful. It certainly does not hurt to meet people who were given death sentences 10 years ago...and are still alive.

• **Have an advocate.** This is someone who accompanies you to all your doctor appointments, takes notes, keeps track of paperwork and argues for you when you're hospitalized.

A good advocate can also research the particular cancer and filter his/her findings to you so you are not overwhelmed by all the information.

• **Get a fax machine.** Having one at home will make it much easier to send, receive and make copies of all your medical records (many fax machines do double duty as a copier).

If you have access to a fax machine at work or someplace else outside your home, think twice before using it. You may not want others to see all your medical records.

• **Make use of the Internet.** You're going to need information and explanations. But if you don't have a computer at home, ask to use a friend's or go to a nearby library, copy shop or cybercafe.

Especially helpful: National Cancer Institute, *www.cancer.gov/newscenter*.

• **Make friends with your doctor's staff.** That way, when you call with a question or problem, they'll treat you as an individual—and make sure you get what you need.

Drop off cookies, flowers or even gift certificates to thank them.

• **Ask your doctor's office to schedule the appointments when you are referred to specialists.** They can line up an appointment sooner than you can.

• **Buy a wig *before* undergoing chemotherapy**—if the drugs to be used are likely to cause hair loss. Your doctor can probably prescribe a wig for you. And that's a good idea because it means that part or even all of the cost might be covered by health insurance.

• **Indulge yourself.** When Kohn took steroids as part of his treatment, he craved fatty foods such as chicken wings and french fries. That's not unusual.

Kohn's wife was horrified. She thought he wasn't taking care of himself. But the food provided one of his few sources of pleasure during this time.

●**If you don't have cable television, get it.** You'll often be too sick to read or write. A funny movie or TV show can do wonders to lift your mood—and it's critical that you keep your spirits up.

●**Plan for depression.** Bloch noted that "everything about cancer is depressing. Expect down days and plan things that cheer you up at those times."

Ask your doctor about antidepressant therapy to ease the feelings of hopelessness that often accompany cancer.

Cancer-Fighting Sprouts

Broccoli sprouts contain the potent cancer-fighting compound called *glucosinolate of sulforaphane* in concentrations 20–50 times higher than those found in "adult" broccoli. One gram (g) of three-day-old sprouts has as much sulforaphane as 25 g of adult broccoli.

Bonus: The sprouts lack the familiar broccoli taste, which many people find objectionable. Broccoli sprouts taste similar to alfalfa sprouts and are good on salads and sandwiches.

Paul Talalay, MD, professor of pharmacology and molecular sciences, Johns Hopkins University School of Medicine, Baltimore.

Use Sunscreen on Fingernails and Toenails

Skin cancer that strikes beneath fingernails and toenails can be prevented by using sunscreen and nail polish. Without protection, two-thirds of the sun's rays penetrate the nail to the nail bed.

Sign of possible skin cancer: One or more brown or black bands running lengthwise in the nail.

Self-defense: When applying sunscreen, cover hands, fingers, toes and nails. Use nail polish. Dark colors provide the most protection. But colorless polish, which can be worn by men, is also effective.

Richard K. Scher, MD, professor of dermatology, University of North Carolina, Chapel Hill.

Eat More Tomatoes

Eating tomatoes helps prevent heart attack and stroke—as well as cancer. The yellow, jelly-like material that surrounds tomato seeds makes blood less "sticky," inhibiting the formation of dangerous blood clots that can trigger heart attack or stroke. Research is under way to develop a clot-busting drug containing *P3*—a compound found in the jellylike material. Such medication could replace or supplement low-dose aspirin as a heart attack and stroke preventive. Until then, heart and stroke patients should eat two to four raw tomatoes a day.

Asim Duttaroy, PhD, professor of nutritional medicine, department of nutrition, University of Oslo, Sweden.

Nuts vs. Cholesterol

Eating moderate amounts of pecans (three-quarters of a cup daily for eight weeks) can lower LDL (bad) cholesterol levels by 10%, a recent study has shown.

The monounsaturated and polyunsaturated fats in the nuts are responsible for this effect, especially when nuts take the place of saturated fats in the diet.

Studies with almonds and walnuts have shown similar results. Nuts also contain high amounts of heart-healthy fiber, vitamin E, copper and magnesium.

Wanda Morgan Eastman, PhD, RD, an associate professor of human nutrition, New Mexico State University, Las Cruces. Her eight-week study was published in the *Journal of the American Dietetic Association,* 360 Park Ave. South, New York, NY 10010.

Possible Ulcer Protection

Vitamin C may be an effective way to prevent ulcers and reduce the risk of gastric cancer. People with high blood levels of ascorbic acid —the chemical name for vitamin C—were less likely to show signs of infection from *Helicobacter pylori,* a common cause of ulcers. Try to get 250 to 500 milligrams of vitamin C daily from foods and supplements.

Good food sources: Oranges, red bell peppers, strawberries.

Joel A. Simon, MD, MPH, FACN, professor of clinical medicine and epidemiology and biostatistics at the University of California San Francisco School of Medicine and staff physician at San Francisco Veterans Affairs Medical Center.

Exercising Before a Fatty Meal Can Save Your Life

Eating fatty foods causes a spike in triglyceride levels. Over time, this surge of triglyceride levels raises heart disease risk.

Recent finding: In men who exercised for an hour before eating a high-fat meal, triglyceride levels rose only 40% as high. Exercising after eating lowered the predicted spikes by only 5%.

Theory: Exercise increases production of enzymes that rapidly clear triglycerides from the blood.

Tom R. Thomas, PhD, professor, department of nutritional sciences at the University of Missouri in Columbia. His study was published in the *Journal of Applied Physiology,* 9650 Rockville Pike, Bethesda, MD 20814.

Snowblowers May Not Be Safer Than Shoveling

Snowblowers are not necessarily the safest alternative to manual shoveling for people at risk for heart attack.

In a recent study of 20 heart attack sufferers who were admitted to a Michigan hospital during a blizzard, three of them were shoveling snow and two were using snowblowers. Both practices can cause a person's heart rate and blood pressure to rise significantly. Snow shoveling has been shown to increase systolic blood pressure (the upper number) to 200—optimal systolic pressure is 120 or below—and snow blowing raises it to 160. If there are atherosclerotic plaques in your arteries, these surges in blood pressure can cause them to rupture, triggering a heart attack.

Self-defense: If you have a history of heart disease or have high blood pressure or other coronary risk factors, consult your physician before removing snow yourself.

Barry A. Franklin, PhD, director, Cardiac Rehabilitation and Exercise Laboratories, William Beaumont Hospital, Royal Oak, MI.

Do You Have Diabetes?

Most people with diabetes don't know they have it until serious complications have already developed. There are some early signs and symptoms of diabetes that you should look out for. *They include...*

- **Blurred vision.**
- **Tingling or numbness in the legs, feet or fingers.**
- **Frequent skin infections.**
- **Recurring infections in your gums and/or urinary tract.**
- **Itching of skin and/or genitals.**
- **Drowsiness.**
- **Slow healing of cuts and bruises.**

Claresa Levetan, MD, chief medical officer, Lankenau Institute of Medical Research, Wynnewood, PA, and a cochair of the committee that revised diabetes prevention guidelines for the American Association of Clinical Endocrinologists.

Diabetes/Pizza Trap

In one study, blood sugar (glucose) levels remained elevated into the next morning in type 1 (insulin-dependent) diabetics who had pizza for dinner. Levels also rose in those who ate a nonpizza meal, but they returned to normal by morning.

Pizza seems to have a unique propensity to raise glucose levels for six to 12 hours.

If you are diabetic: Ask your doctor about taking long-acting insulin before eating pizza—or other Italian dishes, such as manicotti or ravioli, which may also elevate glucose.

Jo Ann Ahern, RN, MSN, coordinator, pediatric program, Yale–New Haven Hospital, New Haven, CT. Her study of diabetics was published in *Diabetes Care*, 6925 E. Tenth St., Indianapolis 46219.

An Itch May Be More Than Skin Deep

When troubled by itching, try to focus on the cause.

Trap: Severe, prolonged itching can indicate disease of the thyroid, kidney or liver…lymphoma…or other problems. If an itch does not go away after a few weeks, be sure to consult your doctor.

To be more comfortable in the meantime: Cool the skin with compresses or nonprescription lotions like Sarna Lotion. Oral antihistamines help relieve itching from allergic reactions—and can be used for sedation if itching keeps you awake. Topical cortisone cream helps inflamed skin. If those don't help, ask your doctor about prescriptions. Ultraviolet light often helps eczema and itching that has no obvious cause.

Neal Schultz, MD, a dermatologist in private practice, 1130 Park Ave., New York City 10128.

Natural Relief for Crohn's Disease and IBS

Peppermint oil relieves the painful cramping brought on by Crohn's disease and irritable bowel syndrome (IBS).

Helpful: Place one drop of the oil in a cup of warm water, add some sugar, if desired, and drink the mixture 15 to 30 minutes before eating—or when symptoms begin.

Warning: Do not consume peppermint oil straight, and stop taking the mixture if it causes heartburn. Peppermint oil can be purchased at most health-food stores.

Tim Koch, MD, director, section of gastroenterology, Washington Hospital Center and Georgetown University School of Medicine, both in Washington, DC.

Knock Out Migraines… Naturally

Alexander Mauskop, MD, director, New York Headache Center in New York City, *www.nyheadache.com*. He is author of *Migraine and Headache.* Oxford American Pain Library.

Twenty-six million Americans suffer from migraines. Fortunately, a drug-free program has been proven in many double-blind clinical trials to bring substantial relief to two-thirds of migraineurs. *The key is the three natural substances that were used in the trials…*

•**Magnesium** opens constricted blood vessels, slows down inflammation and interrupts the action of neurotransmitters that lead to a migraine. Half of migraineurs are deficient in this mineral.

•**Riboflavin** (vitamin B-2) plays a critical role in the proper function of *mitochondria,* the energy generators within cells. Studies have shown that a high dose—400 milligrams (mg) daily—can reduce the severity *and* frequency of migraines.

•**Feverfew** has been used as a folk remedy for centuries. In recent years, four double-blind studies have shown this herb to be more effective than a placebo in preventing migraines. Researchers are uncertain how feverfew works, but it is believed to interrupt the inflammatory process that triggers headaches.

For optimum benefit, I typically advise my patients to take the three natural substances simultaneously—in the daily doses found to be effective in clinical studies…

Magnesium—300 mg…riboflavin—400 mg… and feverfew—100 mg.

This treatment has virtually no side effects. For the best absorption, take half of the daily dose twice a day, with meals.

Important: Magnesium comes in numerous chemical varieties, but magnesium oxide or chelated magnesium works best. Feverfew, like all herbs, varies considerably from one preparation to another. Choose a brand that is recognizable and reliable.

Caution: If you are taking blood thinners or have any allergies to herbs, check with your doctor before starting this regimen.

AN INTEGRATED STRATEGY

The mineral-vitamin-herb combination is most effective if you also…

• **Exercise.** Regular running, biking, rapid walking or similar aerobic workouts—strenuous enough to work up a sweat and increase your pulse substantially—will decrease headache frequency and intensity. Exercise at least four times weekly for 30 minutes or more each time.

• **Avoid "triggers."** Many headaches are provoked by certain foods, drinks or activities.

Biggest offender: Caffeine. Eliminate caffeine-containing drinks and drugs. If you cannot give up coffee entirely, restrict yourself to one cup a day.

Some people also get headaches after drinking alcohol, particularly red wine, brandy, bourbon and dark beer. The same goes for aged cheese and meat products that contain nitrates (bacon, corned beef and pastrami). Eliminate these products, and see if your headaches stop.

• **Get enough sleep.** The average person needs at least seven hours per night. Sleep deprivation can trigger a headache.

• **Schedule quiet time.** Exercise helps to defuse the tension and stress that exacerbate the frequency and intensity of headaches. In addition, make time in your day for whatever else you find relaxing—meditation, reading, family fun, etc.

A Smarter Approach to Chronic Pain

Mark Allen Young, MD, a licensed acupuncturist and chairman of physical medicine and rehabilitation at the Maryland Rehabilitation Center in Baltimore. He is the author of *Women and Pain: Why It Hurts and What You Can Do.* Hyperion. His Web site is *www.drmarkyoung.com.*

If you rely exclusively on aspirin, ibuprofen or another over-the-counter (OTC) medication to control pain, you might be shortchanging yourself.

Few people realize it, but there is often a much more effective way to combat pain. A comprehensive treatment approach, including strategic eating habits, supplements, exercise and medication, will stop pain for a variety of common ailments.

It is best to try different strategies to see what works for you. Before attempting any of these approaches, however, consult your doctor to determine the cause of your pain.

ARTHRITIS

OTC pain-relieving remedies used alone are woefully inadequate for osteoarthritis pain. *Better approaches…*

• **Eat avocados and soy foods,** such as tofu and tempeh. They decrease inflammation and pain, while promoting cartilage growth. Consume these foods daily.

• **Eat more fish.** The fatty acids in cold-water fish, such as salmon, mackerel and tuna, help prevent body chemicals called *prostaglandins* from triggering inflammation. Consume at least three servings weekly.

• **Perform cardiovascular exercise daily.** Swimming and brisk walking are ideal. Both decrease pressure on joints by strengthening surrounding muscles. Vigorous exercise also triggers the release of *endorphins,* the body's natural painkillers.

•**Take glucosamine.** This supplement helps to nourish cartilage and gives it more elasticity. Recent studies show that glucosamine temporarily relieves pain as well as ibuprofen, and it is unlikely to cause any side effects.

Typical dosage: 500 milligrams three times daily.

BACK PAIN

Half of all adult Americans suffer from back pain. More than 90% of these cases involve muscle spasm caused by injury, poor posture or excessive body weight.

If you are experiencing back pain that is accompanied by pain or numbness in the buttocks, legs or feet, see a doctor immediately. These can be symptoms of a more serious condition, such as disk or nerve damage. *But when pain is the only symptom…*

•**Apply a pain-relieving ointment twice daily.** The active ingredient in these products temporarily prevents pain signals from reaching the brain. *Good choices:* ArthroMax, Bengay and Joint-Ritis.

•**Learn to relax.** Stress accentuates your perception of pain…promotes muscle tightness … and increases the risk for injury.

Devote at least 40 minutes daily to meditation, exercise, yoga or another relaxing activity.

•**Stretch and strengthen abdominal and back muscles.** Four times per day, lie on your back with knees slightly bent…tighten muscles in the belly and buttocks…and push the lower back against the floor.

Hold for five seconds, then relax and repeat.

FIBROMYALGIA

This misunderstood and frequently misdiagnosed condition is characterized by widespread, chronic pain involving multiple "tender points" in the upper neck, back, shoulders and hips.

The conventional treatments—such as painkillers, antidepressants, muscle relaxants and the injection of anesthetics—are rarely effective. *Additional options…*

•**Consume apples and/or apple juice.** They contain *malic acid,* a substance that appears to ease fibromyalgia pain. Consume at least two apples or two eight-ounce glasses of juice daily.

•**Try acupuncture.** It triggers a massive release of endorphins, which can reduce pain for more than a week after each treatment.

To locate an acupuncturist in your area, contact the American Academy of Medical Acupuncture at 310-364-0193 or *www.medical acupuncture.org.*

•**Do *not* give up on exercise.** People with fibromyalgia often stop exercising because it's painful. But inactivity weakens muscles and renders them more sensitive to pain. Low-impact aerobic conditioning exercises, such as swimming, stationary bicycling or stretching, are often helpful.

HEADACHE

The vast majority of headaches are *tension headaches,* caused by muscle spasm in the head or neck. OTC pain-relievers can provide temporary relief. *Also important…*

•**Drink more water.** Dehydration is a leading cause of headaches. Consume at least eight eight-ounce glasses of water daily.

•**Avoid caffeine.** It increases muscle tension. Drink no more than one cup of coffee per day.

•**Practice acupressure.** It minimizes pain and stiffness.

What to do: Firmly press your finger or thumb into the hollow between the skull and the back of the neck. Hold for 90 seconds. Repeat three times daily.

•**Take feverfew.** This herb contains *parthenolide,* an agent that reduces spasms in blood vessels in the head. Feverfew works for migraines as well as tension headaches.

MUSCLE STRAIN

This usually involves damage to ligaments, the cords of fibrous tissue that bind bones together. *To reduce pain and speed healing…*

•**Apply ice within 24 hours of the injury** …wrap it with an elastic bandage…and elevate it above heart-level to reduce swelling.

•**Take a hot bath.** Warmth relieves muscle spasm. But try ice first—it's not a good idea to take a hot bath or apply heat within 24 hours of a muscle injury.

●**Take vitamin E.** It blocks the effects of harmful molecules (free radicals) that result from muscle injuries. Check with your doctor for the dose that's right for you.

●**Apply capsaicin cream.** Capsaicin is the potent compound that makes chili peppers hot. The OTC ointment warms the area and reduces pain. Apply twice daily, starting 24 hours after the injury has occurred. Beware that long-term use can deaden nerve endings.

Good choice: Zostrix.

Acupuncture *Really* Works

Gary Kaplan, DO, a clinical associate professor and director of the Kaplan Clinic, Georgetown University School of Medicine in Washington, DC, as well as a physician–acupuncturist in private practice in Arlington, VA. He is a director at large for the Medical Acupuncture Research Foundation in Santa Monica, CA.

Recently, a National Institutes of Health (NIH) panel deemed acupuncture to be "an acceptable alternative, or part of a comprehensive treatment program" for several types of pain, including headache, arthritis, lower back pain, menstrual cramps and carpal tunnel syndrome.

HOW DOES ACUPUNCTURE WORK?

The Chinese believe that acupuncture, a 2,500-year-old practice, works by affecting the energy pathways called "meridians" that run throughout the body.

These meridians are believed to carry "qi" (pronounced *chee*), an energy force that must be in precise balance for good heath.

Poor health habits—getting too little sleep, eating the wrong foods, etc.—cause qi to become unbalanced.

Acupuncture helps rebalance qi by stimulating specific points along these meridians with extremely fine needles.

Medical researchers in the Western world say that acupuncture needles cause the release of endorphins, cortisone and other natural pain-killing and anti-inflammatory agents.

This explanation is backed up by controlled studies demonstrating acupuncture's effect on the nervous system and on hormone levels and immune function.

SAFE AND EFFECTIVE RELIEF

In addition to relieving many kinds of musculoskeletal pain, acupuncture also works well for nausea and vomiting associated with chemotherapy and pregnancy.

It's also effective against asthma, bronchitis, digestion problems and drug addiction.

You might choose acupuncture over pain-killing drugs or other conventional treatments if you are unable to tolerate the side effects of medications.

For anyone who falls into one of these categories, acupuncture can be a godsend.

In one study from Denmark, seven of 28 people scheduled for knee surgery got such effective relief from acupuncture therapy that they were able to cancel their surgeries.

In my own practice, acupuncture has helped many patients who were not helped by drug therapy or other conventional treatments.

In addition, acupuncture is extremely safe. Some patients develop minor bruising at the site of needle insertion, but that doesn't happen often.

Critics of acupuncture have long discussed the risks of contracting hepatitis from a dirty needle. In fact, acupuncture-induced hepatitis is almost unheard of in the US. That's because most practitioners use disposable needles.

UNDERSTANDING THE PROCEDURE

During a typical acupuncture session, the acupuncturist will take a comprehensive history and ask about the patient's sleep patterns, dietary habits, etc. and about any symptoms that he might be experiencing.

As part of the ensuing exam, the patient's pulse is measured several times in different areas of the wrist...and the tongue is checked for discoloration or swelling.

On the basis of this exam, the acupuncturist can pinpoint areas in the body where qi has become stagnant or unbalanced. Needles are placed in a specific combination of points.

FINDING AN ACUPUNCTURIST

There are now more than 10,000 licensed acupuncturists in the US. Roughly 3,000 of these are physicians. The rest are lay practitioners.

It's best to find a physician-acupuncturist. A physician can catch any serious ailment that a lay practitioner might miss. In addition, your health insurance may be more likely to cover acupuncture administered by a physician.

To obtain a referral to a qualified physician–acupuncturist, call the American Academy of Medical Acupuncture at 310-364-0193 or visit *www.medicalacupuncture.org.*

If you decide to work with a lay acupuncturist, make sure he/she is certified by the National Certification Commission for Acupuncture and Oriental Medicine, *www.nccaom.org,* 904-598-1005.

Don't Put Up with Dizziness

Brian W. Blakley, MD, PhD, professor and chair of the department of otolaryngology at the University of Manitoba in Winnipeg, Manitoba, Canada. He is the author of *Feeling Dizzy.* Wiley.

Seventy-six million Americans experience dizzy spells from time to time, and it's the fourth most common reason that people consult a doctor. But few get effective treatment. That's because dizziness is often dismissed as a symptom of a psychological problem, such as anxiety.

If you've ever felt dizzy after standing up too fast, you know that such a spell is harmless and passes in seconds. But other forms of dizziness occur intermittently and have causes that are difficult to identify.*

Here are the primary types of dizziness and how to get help for each…

VERTIGO

The most common type of dizziness, vertigo, is marked by a spinning or whirling sensation

*If dizziness is accompanied by double vision, incontinence, arm and/or leg weakness, difficulty speaking or swallowing or severe headache, see a doctor immediately. These symptoms suggest a life-threatening condition, such as stroke, brain tumor or aneurysm.

16

that occurs while you're standing still. Ear infections are not the only culprit. *Vertigo can also be caused by…*

• **Benign paroxysmal positional vertigo.** BPPV typically results from a blow to the head or age-related degeneration of the vestibular system, made up of the brain and the parts of the inner ears that act as motion sensors.

An attack of BPPV lasts about 15 seconds and occurs when you roll over in bed, look down or turn your head sharply to the left or right.

A careful physician can diagnose BPPV by watching your eye movements as you demonstrate the positions that trigger the vertigo. The condition typically subsides on its own.

• **Ménière's disease.** This condition is associated with an accumulation of fluid in one or both inner ears. It triggers recurrent attacks of dizziness that last for hours…temporary hearing loss in one ear…tinnitus…and/or a feeling of pressure in the ear.

If the problem lasts for more than a week, see an otolaryngologist. He/she should perform an audiogram to evaluate your hearing and an eye test known as *electronystagmography* (ENG). Throughout an ENG exam, cold and warm water are alternately poured into the ear. Eye movements are then recorded and analyzed to determine inner ear function.

To control Ménière's disease, doctors will usually prescribe the antihistamine *meclizine* (Antivert), which suppresses the vestibular system. To decrease fluid accumulation, you may also need to take a diuretic and/or steroids.

The treatment for Ménière's disease typically takes three months. At that point, you should be reevaluated to see if you still need to be on medication.

• **Vestibular neuronitis.** This condition frequently confuses doctors because it mimics influenza. People with vestibular neuronitis suffer from nausea and vomiting as well as sudden vertigo following recovery from a viral infection. It is believed to be caused by an inflammation of the vestibular nerve, which links the brain and inner ear.

An otolaryngologist can diagnose the condition by reviewing your history and performing an ENG exam. Bed rest and medication, such as *meclizine* or, in more severe cases, the sedative *diazepam* (Valium), are the most effective treatments.

MILD TURNING

Mild turning is the most benign variety of dizziness. It causes a sensation that you are slowly turning—either vertically or horizontally—while standing still.

If symptoms are mild and no underlying cause, such as a viral infection or tumor, can be found, no treatment is necessary.

However, if the sensation really bothers you, your doctor should prescribe a sedative, such as diazepam, for one week. Physical therapy also helps.

Important: Because mild turning can be symptomatic of a brain disorder or the result of a "silent" stroke (transient ischemic attack, or TIA), consult a neurologist if you also have problems swallowing or speaking or experience leg or arm weakness.

IMBALANCE

This type of dizziness is common among people who are age 60 or beyond. Imbalance creates a swaying or wobbling sensation or a feeling of lightheadedness. This sensation may make it difficult to walk without falling.

Imbalance is typically caused by age-related degeneration of nerves in the ears. It can also be triggered by diabetes, tranquilizers or anticonvulsants, heart problems, anxiety and/or muscle weakness.

To diagnose imbalance, doctors should perform an audiogram and an ENG exam.

Imbalance is hard to treat. The preferred method is consistent physical activity. Exercise will rehabilitate weakened muscles, improve your balance and train your eyes to move independently of your head.

Helpful exercise for walking imbalance: Stand for 30 seconds with one foot in front of the other, the heel touching the toe. Switch feet, and hold the position for 30 seconds. Repeat three times daily. Perform this exercise in bare feet or in shoes with flat soles.

By increasing levels of the brain chemical *serotonin,* the tricyclic antidepressants, such as *amitriptyline* or *nortriptyline* (Pamelor), may also help. Research has linked serotonin defi-

ciency to dizziness, particularly in people who are depressed or anxious.

Sedatives are not recommended. They can worsen imbalance.

FAINTING

Fainting is commonly caused by the use of blood pressure medication. The less obvious causes include diabetes, dehydration or a viral infection. If a precipitating event cannot be identified or you experience fainting episodes more than once a year, see your physician. Repeated fainting episodes may indicate a cardiovascular or neurological disorder.

To guard against fainting, exercise daily and avoid activities that trigger episodes. This may include getting up from a sitting position too quickly.

To locate a doctor or physical therapist who specializes in dizziness, contact the Vestibular Disorders Association at 800-837-8428 or *www. vestibular.org.*

Natural Strategies for Beating Gum Disease

Victor Zeines, DDS, a dentist in private practice in New York City. Dr. Zeines is the author of *Healthy Mouth, Healthy Body.* Kensington.

If you think losing your teeth is the greatest risk of gum disease, think again. People with gum disease are *three times* more likely to have heart problems and *twice* as likely to have a stroke as individuals who have healthy mouths. Gum disease may also worsen respiratory problems, such as chronic bronchitis.

In addition to brushing at least twice daily and flossing every evening, it helps to use a water irrigator set on low to stimulate blood flow to your gums. This helps fight gum disease.

You have probably been taught to visit a dentist every six months. But a visit every *three* months is often preferable for those with numerous fillings or a personal or family history of gum disease.

Beyond these basic strategies, I also recommend —in addition to a multivitamin—three vitamin and mineral supplements…

•**Vitamin C.** It helps prevent tooth decay and promotes healthy gums.

Daily dosage: 1,000 milligrams (mg), preferably in a time-release form.

•**Calcium.** Your teeth are made mostly of calcium, so you need a good daily supply of this essential mineral.

Daily dosage: 1,500 mg, preferably as calcium gluconate or calcium citrate. Both forms are easily absorbed. Always take with vitamin D.

•**Magnesium.** This mineral works with calcium to build strong teeth. Magnesium also helps to prevent tooth decay and promotes recovery from gum disease.

Daily dosage: 500 mg.

Supplements and checkups won't do much good, though, if your overall diet is poor. A diet that produces an acidic environment in your mouth leads to tooth decay and gum disease.

Culprits: Foods that contain lots of sugar, fat and/or protein.

Self-defense: Eat more fresh fruits and vegetables and fewer processed foods. Fruits and vegetables promote an alkaline environment in the mouth. They are also high in fiber, which helps clean the mouth.

RINSING FOR ORAL HEALTH

Bacteria in your mouth are the cause of gum disease and tooth decay. An herbal mouth rinse containing natural antibiotics is especially effective at preventing these problems.

The herbs goldenseal, myrrh and calendula have been used for centuries to improve dental health.

Purchase each herb separately in tincture form, then combine 30 drops of each in a small brown bottle. Store the tincture in a cool, dark place away from children.

Ideally, you should use a water irrigator for the herbal mouth rinse. It allows you to irrigate the pockets between teeth and gums, where bacteria accumulate.

Good choices: Waterpik or any other brand with an irrigation tip that reaches below the gum line.

Cost: About $40 to $80.*

Add one-quarter teaspoon of the herbal mixture to the reservoir of the water jet. After each brushing, spray between each tooth for five seconds.

If you're not using an irrigator, swish for 30 seconds, then spit.

BANISHING BAD BREATH

Careful oral hygiene and rinsing almost always eliminate bad breath. When they fail to do so, I ask my patients if they experience digestive problems, such as heartburn, indigestion or gas. If so, I send them to their doctor for an evaluation.

To determine if poor digestion is causing bad breath, look at your tongue in the mirror. It should be pink. *If your tongue is…*

•**Whitish,** you may be suffering from an infection or virus.

•**Yellowish,** you could have liver or gallbladder problems.

•**Grayish-green,** a stomach or intestinal disorder could be the source of trouble.

Consult your physician if you notice any tongue abnormalities.

CLEARING UP COLD SORES

Cold sores (fever blisters) also threaten your oral health. Caused by *herpes simplex* virus 1, cold sores plague millions of Americans.

Some people are naturally immune to the virus, but almost half of all Americans get cold sores on their lips, gums, tongue or cheeks at least occasionally.

Stress—from illness, poor nutrition or life events—weakens immune function. This makes you more vulnerable to a cold sore outbreak.

Eating fruits and vegetables should help. In addition, stay away from caffeine, alcohol and other substances that weaken the immune system. Some studies suggest that chocolate, peanut butter and nuts can also trigger cold sores.

Some over-the-counter supplements help fight cold sores…

•**Lysine.** Take this amino acid in supplement form or use a cream.

Typical dosage: 500 mg three times a day …or apply cream as directed on the label.

*All prices subject to change.

- **Vitamin C.** It helps block the growth of the herpes virus.

   Typical dosage: 500 mg up to four times a day. Use less if it upsets your stomach.

- **Vitamin B-complex.** Add a B-complex supplement to strengthen the immune system.

   Typical dosage: 100 mg three times a day.

- **Acidophilus.** Take this friendly bacterium to help fight the growth of the herpes virus. Follow label directions as to dosage.

- **Garlic.** Use this as a supplement to help boost immunity.

   Typical dosage: 1 gram tablet daily...or eat raw or cooked garlic daily.

Help for Canker Sores

Canker sores may be aggravated by *sodium lauryl sulfate* (SLS), a detergent found in many toothpaste brands, according to research. SLS is thought to worsen these painful ulcerations by drying out the mouth's protective layer of mucus.

Helpful: Switch to an SLS-free toothpaste brand, such as Rembrandt Natural or Arm & Hammer Tooth Powder.

Kenneth Burrell, DDS, former senior director, council on scientific affairs, American Dental Association, Chicago.

Best Way to Store a Toothbrush

Storing toothbrushes properly stops bacterial growth. Brushes left to air-dry show significantly less bacterial growth the next day than those stored in airtight containers.

Reason: Capping provides a moist environment in which bacteria thrive.

Kaaren Vargas, DDS, PhD, associate professor, department of pediatric dentistry, College of Dentistry, The University of Iowa, Iowa City.

Cataract Danger

Researchers analyzed dietary and eye data for 3,377 people ages 60 to 80 over eight years.

Result: People who ate more white bread, sugary foods and other foods high on the glycemic index (GI)—a measurement of how quickly a food boosts blood sugar levels—were 29% more likely to develop cataracts than those who consumed less of these foods.

Theory: High-GI foods damage the eye lens by exposing the tissues to higher sugar levels than low-GI foods do.

Chung-Jung Chiu, PhD, assistant professor of ophthalmology, Tufts University School of Medicine, Boston.

Protect Yourself Against Indoor Air Pollution

Timothy McCall, MD, a board-certified internist in Oakland, California, medical editor of *Yoga Journal* and author of *Yoga As Medicine*. Bantam. Dr. McCall leads workshops and retreats on yoga and yoga therapy around the country and worldwide. *www.drmccall.com.*

Air pollution is often thought of as an outdoor problem. But a bigger danger may be the toxic air inside our own homes. Indoor levels of various pollutants run two to five times—and sometimes more than 100 times—higher than outdoor levels, according to the Environmental Protection Agency (EPA). This is troublesome because Americans spend the vast majority of their time indoors.

Besides increasing the risk for asthma and cancer, indoor air pollution can cause headaches, burning eyes, nausea, fatigue and other problems. Ironically, the newer fixed-window buildings—designed to improve energy efficiency—exacerbate the problem by trapping stale air inside.

Probably the most immediate danger comes from carbon monoxide. High levels of this colorless, odorless gas—generated by furnaces, water heaters and blocked chimneys—can kill in minutes.

Dishwashers and washing machines release "aerosolized" toxins from the water supply. Tiny particles emitted during cooking—frying and sautéing, in particular—can contribute to asthma and other lung problems.

Home-office equipment—such as printers, copiers and even colored markers—emit toxic chemicals, including toner and solvents. The risk is even greater in small offices that have poor ventilation.

Here's how to reduce your risk of getting sick—or worse—from indoor air pollution…

•**Declare your home smoke-free.** Cigarettes —and especially cigars—leave a toxic residue in the air. This contributes to asthma, lung cancer and children's ear infections.

•**Purchase a carbon monoxide detector.** These are available in the hardware stores for $20 and up.* Have any gas-burning appliances and chimneys checked yearly. And never warm up a car in a closed garage.

•**Test your house for radon.** This naturally occurring and odorless radioactive gas is second only to smoking as a cause of lung cancer. All homes and apartments below the third floor should be tested. Test kits are sold in hardware stores for $20 and up. For questions about radon, contact the National Radon Hotline, 800-767-7236.

•**Consider purchasing air-purifying systems.** Exhaust fans in the kitchen, bathroom, home office and workshop are all advisable. Or open a window and point a fan outward to ventilate a room.

High-efficiency particulate-arresting (HEPA) filters remove cigarette smoke and harmful particulates. Dehumidifiers eliminate excess moisture that leads to the buildup of allergy-causing mold and dust mites. Carbon filters attached to waterlines reduce aerosolized pollutants.

•**Watch out for other sources of in-home pollution.** New carpets, particleboard, plywood and many paints can give off toxic fumes. Hardwood or linoleum flooring and washable throw rugs may be safer alternatives. Scented candles have been shown to give off lead, mercury and other toxins. The beeswax candles are safer. Cedar chips are a safe alternative to mothballs.

•**Air out your house.** On particularly polluted days, I try to keep the windows to my house closed up. Late in the evening, I open them and put on fans to remove the stale air. Similarly, after I have used my laser printer, I open the windows, run the fan and spend the next half hour or so in another room.

•**Fill your house with plants.** Philodendra and spider plants, among others, help purify the air and liven up the decor.

Caught Dirty-Handed

Rebecca Shannonhouse, editor, *Bottom Line/Health*, 281 Tresser Blvd., Stamford, CT 06901.

According to a survey by the American Society for Microbiology, 95% of us *say* we wash our hands after using the restroom—but only 67% of us actually do it.

We all know that washing up after a restroom stop and before preparing food or eating is one of the best ways to curb the spread of disease. It's also a good precaution to take after handling money, coughing, sneezing or touching a pet.

Elaine Larson, RN, PhD, associate dean for research at the Columbia University School of Nursing in New York City, and editor of the *American Journal of Infection Control* provided a primer on how to wash. *Her suggestions…*

•**Use plain soap and water.** This rinses most germs off your hands. But if you've had contact with a person who has an infection, a waterless, alcohol-based, hand-sanitizing gel is probably a better bet. It will kill bacteria more effectively than antibacterial soaps.

•**Don't forget the fingertips.** Most people don't wash their entire hands. Soap and rinse or apply gel to *all* areas of your hand, including the fingertips and under the fingernails.

•**Apply hand lotion.** It helps to prevent dried or cracked skin, which can harbor dangerous infectious agents, such as *gram-negative bacteria* and *Staphylococcus aureus*.

*All prices subject to change.

By the way, screw-cap bottles—and pour spouts—can be problematic. If you pour too much liquid into your palm and return the excess, bacteria from your hands will go back into the container. The soap then becomes contaminated for future washes.

Home Remedy for Liver Spots

Liver spots (age spots) are harmless areas of discoloration caused by excessive sun exposure. If you don't want to purchase lightening creams, you might try a simple home remedy. Mix one teaspoon of grated horseradish root, one-half teaspoon fresh lemon juice, one-half teaspoon vinegar and three drops of rosemary essential oil. With a cotton swab, dab the mixture onto the age spots twice a day, less often if you have sensitive skin. The mildly irritating ingredients will gently exfoliate the top layer of skin, which lightens the spots.

Important: If the spots are dark brown, black, red, white or blue or irregular in size, shape or color, see your dermatologist.

Jeanette Jacknin, MD, a dermatologist in private practice in Scottsdale, AZ, and the author of *Smart Medicine for Your Skin*. Avery.

Getting Help for Embarrassing Medical Problems

Margaret Stearn, MD, a physician who practices general medicine in Oxford, England, with a special interest in diabetes and urologic medicine. Dr. Stearn is a Fellow of the Royal College of Physicians and the author of *Embarrassing Medical Problems: Everything You Always Wanted to Know But Were Afraid to Ask Your Doctor.* Hatherleigh Press.

If you suffer from a backache or dizziness, it's easy to tell your doctor. But what about those nagging symptoms that you are too embarrassed to discuss?

Unfortunately, many patients deprive themselves of effective treatment and, in some cases, endanger their long-term health by failing to disclose certain medical problems. *How to get some help...*

BAD BREATH

Saliva production diminishes during sleep, allowing food debris to stagnate in the mouth. Bacteria break down these residues, producing an unpleasant smell. That's why almost everyone has bad breath (halitosis) upon waking up. It usually disappears after you brush your teeth.

To determine if you have bad breath: Lick the inside of your wrist, wait four seconds, then smell.

Persistent halitosis is generally caused by gum disease (gingivitis). If your gums bleed when you brush your teeth, you most likely have gum disease and, as a result, bad breath. *What to do...*

•**See your dentist** for a checkup and thorough cleaning.

•**Brush your teeth at least twice daily.**

Best method: Clean teeth two at a time for six seconds, moving the brush in a small circular motion while angling it toward the gum.

Or consider buying a battery-powered toothbrush, which often controls gum disease better than manual brushing.

Cost: $10 to $120.*

•**Clean the back of your tongue,** where bacteria accumulate. Use your toothbrush or a tongue scraper.

•**Use an antibacterial mouthwash,** such as Biotène, Cepacol or Listerine Antiseptic.

•**Floss nightly**—especially the molars.

If halitosis persists: See your doctor.

EXCESSIVE PERSPIRATION

Perspiration itself is not smelly, but it is a breeding ground for bacteria that will quickly break down into malodorous fatty acids.

Excessive perspiration (hyperhidrosis) could affect armpits, feet or palms. *What to do...*

•**Armpits.** Women and men should shave their armpits to reduce bacterial buildup. Also switch to an antiperspirant with an active ingredient different from what you're currently using.

*All prices subject to change.

21

•**Feet.** Wear clean, loose-fitting socks made from wool or cotton and at least 30% man-made fiber, such as nylon or polyester. Wash socks in hot water to kill bacteria.

Avoid shoes that are made from synthetic materials. They trap moisture, which enables bacteria to multiply. This is also true for sneakers, so don't wear them for more than four hours a day.

Bathe your feet daily in warm water that contains about 10 drops of tea tree oil per pint of water. This solution has antibacterial properties. Also, use a pumice stone to remove hardened, dead skin from your heels and soles.

•**Palms.** Rub your palms every few hours with an astringent oil, such as cypress or geranium. These essential oils, which are available at health-food stores, can be added to almond oil or a lotion.

If self-treatment doesn't help: Discuss with your doctor. He may prescribe a *20% aluminum chloride* solution or an anticholinergic drug, such as *propantheline* (Pro-Banthine), to reduce the perspiration.

Botulinum toxin (Botox) injections are also a treatment option for severe hyperhidrosis.

As a last resort, surgical division of the sympathetic nerves that cause sweating is almost 100% effective for feet and palms and about 40% effective for armpits.

FEMININE ITCHING

Itching of the vulva (vulval pruritis) is usually caused by a vaginal yeast infection. *What to do...*

•**Try an over-the-counter cream,** such as *butoconazole* (Gyne-Lotrimin) or *miconazole* (Monistat 3). If this doesn't help within a few days, your physician may then recommend a prescription medication, such as *fluconazole* (Diflucan).

Other possible causes include eczema, psoriasis or an allergy.

To relieve the itch: Soak in warm water that contains two handfuls of Epsom salts or ordinary kitchen salt...or dip a washcloth into a salt-water solution and apply to the affected area for relief.

•**Wash only with unscented cleansers,** such as Dove Unscented Beauty Bar or Neutrogena Transparent Dry Skin Formula Fragrance Free. When shampooing your hair, don't let the foam touch your vulva.

•**Don't use feminine deodorants** or apply deodorant or perfume to sanitary pads...wash your underwear with an enzyme-free, perfume-free detergent formulated for sensitive skin... don't use fabric softener...and don't swim in chlorinated water.

FLATULENCE

It's normal to have some gas. Air swallowed during eating typically collects in the stomach and is passed via belching.

Bacteria also cause certain foods, especially beans, to break down into hydrogen, methane and carbon dioxide.

Most people will experience gas (flatulence) more than 10 times a day. *What to do...*

•**Avoid eating large quantities of gas-causing foods at one time.** These include beans, peas, broccoli, cauliflower, artichokes, cabbage, raisins, prunes and apples. They contain hard-to-digest carbohydrates that ferment in the bowels.

Foods that don't cause flatulence: Potatoes, rice, corn and wheat.

•**Avoid carbonated beverages.**

•**Take your time while eating.** Don't rush when you eat...put your fork down between bites...and be sure to chew food thoroughly.

•**Don't chew gum.**

Over-the-counter antiflatulence aids—such as Beano, charcoal tablets, Gas-X or Phazyme —can also relieve flatulence.

JOCK ITCH

Jock itch (*tinea cruris*) causes an itchy, red rash in a man's groin area. The rash is triggered by the same fungus that causes athlete's foot. In fact, it's often "caught" from your own feet. *What to do...*

•**Try an over-the-counter antifungal ointment,** such as *tolnaftate* (Tinactin). If this does not help, consult your doctor.

•**Wear loose, 100% cotton underwear.**

•**Wash with unscented soap,** and dry the groin area carefully after bathing.

•**Wash underwear with an enzyme-free,** perfume-free detergent.

How to Keep Your Mind Sharp at Any Age

Guy McKhann, MD, professor of neurology and neuroscience, Johns Hopkins School of Medicine, and founding director of the Zanvyl Krieger Mind/Brain Institute at Johns Hopkins, both in Baltimore. He is also coauthor, with his spouse, Marilyn Albert, PhD, of *Keep Your Brain Young: The Complete Guide to Physical and Emotional Health and Longevity.* Wiley.

Who hasn't had a "senior moment"—when you find yourself groping for the name of an acquaintance—and worry that it may be a sign of mental decline, or even Alzheimer's?

While the majority of healthy older people can expect changes in their brain and memory function, it does not mean you are losing your faculties.

Here are several ways to keep your brain functioning well…

ADAPT TO CHANGES

Older people often take longer to learn things and also have more trouble remembering, especially when they're tired or under stress.

The good news: Studies show that older people take in and retain new information just as well as those decades younger—provided they take the time to learn it well. In other words, though older people may think they're forgetting things more easily, the reality is that they're not learning them as well in the first place.

Names and phone numbers are among the most difficult things to learn and remember because they tend to be entirely arbitrary.

To improve your memory for new pieces of information…

•**Concentrate** completely on the new information as you're taking it in. Reinforce it by repeating it aloud.

•**Write down** key information as you get it.

•**Break up long lists** of names, numbers or grocery items into separate chunks of five to seven items.

•**Create a mental picture** of what you're trying to remember.

•**Make associations.** Attach a name with a rhyming word or phrase or action, or join it to a color or important occasion.

Example: If you want to remember to call someone when you get home, imagine that you are inserting your door key into a telephone instead of a lock.

Or try this classic politician's trick. When meeting new people, mentally link their name to their home town or state and their profession—so that John becomes "John the automobile dealer from Colorado."

This strategy works because memory is embedded within many different connections in the brain. The more associations you make to new information, the more brain pathways are involved, and the more likely you are to retrieve the information later.

STAY MENTALLY ACTIVE

In one study, our research group selected 1,200 high-performing individuals between the ages of 70 and 80 and tracked them for 10 years. Those who maintained all of their mental abilities engaged in daily activities that exercised their brains in challenging ways. *These activities included…*

•**Reading books.**
•**Doing crossword puzzles.**
•**Using a computer.**
•**Playing a musical instrument.**
•**Attending lectures or concerts.**

You can also do specific exercises (dubbed "neurobics") to stimulate your brain. One of the best books on this subject is *Keep Your Brain Alive: 83 Neurobic Exercises* by the late Lawrence Katz, a noted brain scientist at Duke University.

MINIMIZE TV TIME

The group whose minds stayed sharpest also spent the least time watching television. Watching TV puts the brain in a passive mode, which is less stimulating than active thinking.

STAY PHYSICALLY ACTIVE

Another common factor among the group who maintained their mental capacity is that they did some physical activity every day—walking, riding a bicycle or stationary bike, swimming laps, lifting weights at home or walking up and down stairs.

Other research has found that daily exercise helps sharpen cognitive skills, lift depression and ward off the changes in memory associated with age. Daily exercise has also been linked to lower incidence of dementia and Alzheimer's.

STAY INVOLVED

The final factor common to the people in our study who maintained their mental abilities was a sense of effectiveness. They felt in control of their lives and that they had something to contribute to their family and society.

Supportive relationships can provide proven neurological advantages. For example, studies with rats have shown that an enriched environment, including interaction with other rats, strengthens the connections between existing nerve cells in the hippocampus and increases production of new nerve cells.

CONSIDER VITAMIN E

Vitamin E is a powerful antioxidant. It mops up "free radicals" formed in the brain by the oxidation process, which otherwise stick to the brain's nerve cells, damaging and killing them.

Studies show that taking vitamin E delays the onset of Alzheimer's disease, and might even slow its progression. It also may lower the risk of Parkinson's disease and other degenerative ailments.

It's not clear yet whether vitamin E can actually prevent such diseases or how it may benefit healthy people. Studies are now under way to research these questions. Check with your doctor before starting a vitamin E regimen.

CONSIDER OTHER SUPPLEMENTS

There is no strong evidence for the benefits of these substances, but more studies are currently being conducted with each...

• **Vitamin C** is another powerful antioxidant, with similar benefits to vitamin E.

Recommended dose: 300 milligrams.

• **Coenzyme Q10** helps maintain healthy mitochondria, the tiny packets of enzymes that produce energy in all cells, including the brain's. It also may prevent or slow the progression of Parkinson's.

• **Ginkgo biloba** seems to have a modest benefit for people who have moderate-to-severe Alzheimer's, according to some studies. Because ginkgo biloba thins the blood, it should not be taken with other blood thinners, such as aspirin or *warfarin* (Coumadin), or before undergoing surgery.

Recommended: Talk to your doctor before adding any supplement to your daily regimen.

An Easy Way to Feel More Energetic

If you are over age 40, fatigue is likely to be a frequent complaint. And if you're like many people, your doctor has checked you over and proclaimed that you're fine.

If you get adequate sleep, eat well and generally take good care of yourself, you might try de-cluttering your house and/or work space. Living in a mess—and feeling guilty about it—can be extremely tiring. Clutter also distracts the mind, making it more difficult to concentrate.

Helpful: Try to get one room—or even just one particular area—better organized. You'll get a noticeable boost.

Jamison Starbuck, ND, a naturopathic physician in family practice in Missoula, Montana. She is a past president of the American Association of Naturopathic Physicians and a contributing editor to *The Alternative Advisor: The Complete Guide to Natural Therapies and Alternative Treatments.* Time Life.

Often Overlooked Causes Of Chronic Fatigue

Ronald L. Hoffman, MD, director of the Hoffman Center for Holistic Medicine, located in New York City, *www. drhoffman.com.* He is the author of *Tired All the Time: How to Regain Your Lost Energy.* Pocket Books.

If you feel tired all the time, you have lots of company. Each year, Americans make 500 million visits to the doctor seeking treatment for fatigue.

Many people who frequently feel tired fear they have the debilitating condition *chronic fatigue and immune dysfunction syndrome* (CFIDS).

If your fatigue has persisted for more than six months or it is accompanied by sleep disturbances, joint pain, headaches, inability to concentrate or short-term memory loss, you may indeed have CFIDS.

In such cases, it is best to seek treatment from a CFIDS specialist. For a list of specialists in your area, contact the CFIDS Association of America, Box 220398, Charlotte, North Carolina 28222, 704-365-2343, *www.cfids.org.*

Good news: Only about 10% of my patients with fatigue actually have CFIDS. The rest are suffering from "garden variety" fatigue, caused by too little sleep or exercise, poor dietary habits or other easily correctable problems.

THYROID PROBLEMS

Many cases of chronic fatigue are caused by over- or underproduction of thyroxine. That's the thyroid hormone responsible for regulating how energy is consumed by the body's cells.

Overactive thyroid: Symptoms of hyperthyroidism include fatigue, anxiety, insomnia, weight loss, heat intolerance, heart palpitations and bulging eyes. This condition is treated with the thyroxine-blocking drugs…or with surgery or radioactive iodine to destroy the thyroid gland.

Underactive thyroid: Suspect hypothyroidism if you feel depressed or lethargic, chill easily, are gaining weight or suffer from premenstrual syndrome (PMS), muscle aches, dry skin, eczema, hair loss, low libido, a hoarse throat or frequent colds or flu.

If you're experiencing any of these symptoms, check your basal body temperature. Insert a thermometer under your armpit as soon as you awaken, before getting out of bed. Record results for three consecutive mornings.

An average basal temperature of 97.4°F or lower suggests hypothyroidism. Your doctor can give you a blood test to confirm or negate your suspicions.

Most doctors treat hypothyroidism with synthetic thyroxine (*synthroid*). However, some patients show more improvement when they take *natural* thyroid hormone (derived from beef or pork).

If synthroid doesn't relieve your symptoms, ask your doctor to consider that alternative.

ADRENAL INSUFFICIENCY

Anyone whose fatigue is accompanied by malaise, frequent illness, allergies, low blood pressure or low blood sugar may be making too little of the adrenal hormone *dehydroepiandrosterone* (DHEA).

Adrenal insufficiency is usually caused by autoimmune disease…or by adrenal gland damage stemming from long-term use of cortisone.

If a blood test reveals low levels of DHEA, you might need to take it in pill form.

In Europe, DHEA has long been used to boost immune function and combat fatigue—though few American doctors have much experience with the drug.

To locate an endocrinologist familiar with DHEA, contact the American College for Advancement in Medicine, *www.acam.org.*

DIABETES

Adult-onset diabetes is an often-overlooked source of persistent fatigue. To rule out this condition, ask your doctor for a *fasting blood glucose test.*

The normal range of insulin is 80 to 100 milligrams per deciliter (mg/dL) of blood. If you fall above that range, eating a special diet and getting regular exercise can help lower blood sugar levels. That should boost your energy.

HORMONAL PROBLEMS

In men, some cases of chronic fatigue are caused by abnormally low levels of testosterone. Men who suffer from this problem (which can be spotted with a simple blood test) can boost their energy levels by taking testosterone supplements.

Hormone problems can bring on fatigue in women as well. But tests for hormone imbalances in women are often inaccurate.

Instead of relying on a blood test, women should suspect hormone problems if…

• **Their fatigue is cyclical,** getting worse prior to menstruation and improving afterward.

• **They experience weight gain** of more than five pounds prior to each period.

• **They perpetually crave sugar,** chocolate or spicy foods.

• **They experience migraines** or breast tenderness when taking birth-control pills.

To treat hormone-related fatigue, women should reduce their consumption of alcohol, meat and dairy products…consume more dietary fiber and less sugar and refined foods…take supplements of *gamma linolenic acid* (GLA). It is found in primrose oil, borage oil and black currant seed oil—available at health-food stores. Or consider trying oral contraceptive pills or Zoloft.

Women with *extreme* PMS-related fatigue can ask their doctor about having a *Myers' cocktail* once a month. That is an intravenous drip containing calcium, magnesium and vitamins B and C.

FOOD ALLERGIES

Chronic, mild food allergies can cause fatigue. Suspect allergies if you have dark circles under your eyes…are irritable…depressed…or have frequent infections or dry skin.

Cravings for particular foods or cycles of energy and fatigue also suggest food allergies—especially to wheat and dairy products. These foods can cause the body to produce an energy-sapping morphine-like substance.

Consider a medically supervised fast of one to four days, to see if your energy increases. Add foods back to your diet only with the doctor's permission.

ENVIRONMENTAL TOXINS

If you can't find another source of fatigue, you may be suffering from exposure to indoor pollutants. *Usual culprits…*

- **Benzene.** In linoleum and degreasers.
- **Formaldehyde.** In carpets and drapes.
- **Lead.** In tap water and house paint.
- **Mercury.** In dental fillings and in some house paints.
- **Nitrogen dioxide.** Released by kerosene heaters, gas stoves and furnaces.
- **Trichloroethylene.** Used in dry cleaning.

Have your home tested for environmental toxins. For companies that test air and water, look under "Laboratories–Testing"—in the Yellow Pages.

If toxins *are* a problem, you should consider installing carbon-based water and air filters. Make sure your home is well-ventilated so that fumes can escape. Also, fill your home with house plants to help filter the air.

Your physician should test your blood for chemical markers of contaminants…and your hair for lead, mercury and other toxic metals. If any traces of toxins are found, ask him/her about introducing selenium, vitamin E, beta-carotene, garlic and sodium alginate to your diet. They help rid the body of toxic metals.

For in-depth information on environmental toxins, contact the Human Ecology Action League (HEAL), Box 509, Stockbridge, GA 30281, *www. healnatl.org.*

THE ROLE OF SUGAR

In many cases, fatigue is the result of eating too much sugar. Sugar and refined carbohydrates make your blood sugar rise. This signals the pancreas to produce insulin. Too much insulin leads to *hypoglycemia* (or low blood sugar), which causes extreme fatigue.

If you suspect hypoglycemia, ask your doctor for an oral *glucose-tolerance* test. If, during this test, you experience any heart palpitations, mental confusion or extreme fatigue, or feel dizzy or shaky, suspect a sugar problem—even if your doctor says your blood sugar levels are normal. Treatment is simple—stop eating sugar.

Also helpful: Eating six small meals instead of the usual three big meals. Small, frequent meals help stabilize blood sugar levels.

Finally, ask your doctor about taking ergogenic (energy-generating) dietary supplements, including vitamin B-15…L-carnitine…octacosanol, a wheat germ extract…ginseng.

Bedtime Trick

Wearing a fresh pair of socks to bed helps you fall asleep faster by stabilizing your core body temperature.

But avoid 100% cotton socks, which tend to absorb moisture. Instead, choose acrylic, polyester, polypropylene and the cotton-synthetic blends that wick away moisture.

Nicholas Romansky, DPM, a podiatrist in Media, PA. He treats the US World Cup and Olympic soccer teams for foot and ankle injuries.

Surprising Ways to Shed Unwanted Pounds Easily

Stephanie Dalvit-McPhillips, PhD, a registered dietitian with a doctorate in nutritional biochemistry. She maintains a private counseling practice in Willoughby, OH, where she treats people with weight problems and eating disorders. Dr. Dalvit-McPhillips is the author of *The Right Bite: Outsmart 43 Scientifically Proven Fat Triggers and Beat the Dieter's Curse.* Fair Winds.

If you've tried every fad diet but failed to reach your ideal weight, stop blaming yourself. No single diet can address all the complex factors that contribute to weight gain.

In two decades of nutrition research and clinical practice, I've identified dozens of hidden triggers that can cause weight gain—in some cases, *even when you don't overeat.*

Some triggers alter your metabolism, causing you to burn fat and calories inefficiently. Others spark irresistible cravings that give way to out-of-control bingeing.

The key is to identify and avoid your personal triggers. *Here are eight that may surprise you...*

SENSORY CUES

Have you ever claimed to gain weight just by looking at food? Well, you may be right.

In a recent Yale University study, insulin levels skyrocketed in hungry individuals exposed to the sight, smell and even the mere mention of charcoal-broiled steaks. Participants' bodies started converting glucose to fat even before they had taken their first bite.

What to do: Don't linger near buffet tables or dessert trays—especially if you are hungry.

LACK OF FIBER

Low-fiber diets typically provide a lot of fat and calories but few nutrients. Such diets also lack bulk, which means you need to eat more to feel full.

The high-fiber foods are filling, nutritionally dense and relatively low in fat and refined sugar. High-fiber foods also help to stabilize blood glucose and insulin levels.

What to do: Get at least 25 grams of fiber in your daily diet. Good resources include whole grains, fruits, vegetables and legumes.

INSUFFICIENT CALORIES

When you limit calories to 1,000 or fewer daily, your body starts to pilfer protein from lean body tissue, destroying the muscle mass necessary to burn fat and calories. You also begin to produce an overabundance of *lipoprotein lipase,* an enzyme that stores fat in your cells.

You may lose a lot of weight on a very low-calorie diet. But once you resume eating normally, your body will convert what it now perceives as excess calories into fat.

What to do: Do not eat fewer than 1,400 calories daily. Total calories should be divided among several meals and snacks.

DIET FOODS

You may assume that you can eat more if foods are labeled "low-fat" or "lite." Wrong. Despite the catchy labeling, these foods can be packed with sugar and calories. "Sugar-free" products may contain aspartame or saccharin—sweeter-than-sugar substitutes that can provoke a sweet tooth.

What to do: Read ingredient and nutrition labels. Avoid foods that derive more than 20% of calories from fat. And don't over-indulge in low-fat goodies.

SALT AND FLAVOR ENHANCERS

Scientists aren't sure why salt triggers compulsive eating. It may trigger certain hormonal changes that amplify hunger, or we may eat more of the foods we find flavorful.

In addition to salt, the food manufacturers can choose from more than 2,000 flavor enhancers to make packaged snacks and meals irresistible. But many of these ingredients, such as monosodium glutamate and ammonium carbonate, may cause you to not only eat more, but also to store more of what you do eat as fat.

What to do: Avoid salt and foods with artificial flavor-boosters. Use lemon, herbs, balsamic vinegar and no-salt substitutes.

THIRST

People frequently confuse thirst for hunger. What's more, we neglect to count the calories we drink. For example, most 12-ounce sodas contain 150 calories.

27

What to do: Before surrendering to cravings, drink a glass of water—then reassess your hunger. When choosing beverages, stick to water or herbal tea.

CAFFEINE AND NICOTINE

Often trumpeted as appetite suppressants, caffeine and nicotine actually *increase* hunger and cravings in certain individuals.

Both substances trigger our fight-or-flight response, which causes glucose to flood into the bloodstream, providing quick energy and temporarily suppressing the appetite. But as blood glucose levels rise, so do insulin levels.

Result: Within one hour of consuming caffeine (even as little as one cup of coffee) or nicotine, glucose levels nosedive. This leaves you ravenous.

Especially worrisome: Secondhand smoke. People exposed to smoke experience the same fluctuations in their blood sugar, but—unlike a smoker—won't light up when they feel hunger.

What to do: Avoid caffeine for three months. Are you able to forgo that midmorning donut? Have you shed pounds? If so, caffeine is a trigger to be avoided. Nicotine should be eliminated—weight-gain trigger or not. Talk to your doctor about quitting smoking...and avoid secondhand smoke whenever possible.

NOT ENOUGH SLEEP

Sleep-deprived people may increase their daily calorie consumption by as much as 15%, according to research conducted at Emory University School of Medicine in Atlanta.

What to do: Strive to get eight hours of sleep every night.

Super Fat-Blocker

Arnold Fox, MD, an internist and cardiologist in private practice in Beverly Hills, CA. He is coauthor of *The Fat Blocker Diet: The Revolutionary Discovery That Lowers Cholesterol, Reduces Fat, and Controls Weight Naturally.* St. Martin's Press.

In my many years of practicing medicine, I've seen every kind of diet aid you can imagine. But when it comes to producing lasting weight loss, I've never seen anything like *chitosan* (pronounced KITE-o-san).

This natural food supplement—made from the shells of lobsters—forms a gel in the stomach. This gel bonds with any fats that are present, forming fatty "clumps" that are indigestible. These clumps pass out of the body in the feces.

Animal studies have shown that chitosan taken before a meal blocks absorption of up to 50% of consumed fat. Chitosan can combine 8 to 10 times its own weight in fat.

One double-blind study published in Italy found that people who ate a low-fat diet and used chitosan lost an average of 16 pounds... compared with seven pounds for those who followed a low-fat diet without chitosan.

I usually tell my overweight patients to set a target weight, then take 1,000 milligrams of chitosan 30 minutes before eating lunch and dinner. Once the goal is reached, they can stop taking the chitosan.

Taking chitosan does *not* give you permission to eat whatever you want. But it will give you an extra push in the right direction.

There's no evidence that chitosan causes any side effects—but consult your doctor before trying it.

Caution: Avoid chitosan if you're allergic to shellfish, or are pregnant or breast-feeding. Don't take vitamins A, D or E within four hours of taking chitosan. If you do, the health benefits of these vitamins will be lost.

Chitosan pills are available at most drugstores.

Calcium Can Help You Lose Weight

If you don't consume enough calcium, your body overproduces *calcitriol*. Scientists at the University of Tennessee recently discovered that this hormone promotes fat storage in the body.

To verify these findings, researchers analyzed the calcium intake and weight levels of more than 10,000 Americans. People with an average intake of 255 milligrams (mg) a day were 75%

more likely to be overweight than those with an average intake of 1,350 mg a day.

Important: Dieters who get calcium from dairy products lose more weight than those who get calcium from supplements. Based on these findings, dieters should get four daily servings of nonfat or low-fat dairy products, which supply about 1,300 mg of calcium.

Barbara Levine, PhD, RD, associate clinical professor of nutrition in medicine, Weill Cornell Medical College in New York City.

The Right Equipment For Walking

Marilyn L. Bach, PhD, a certified personal trainer and fitness consultant in St. Paul, MN. She is the coauthor of ShapeWalking: Six Easy Steps to Your Best Body. *Hunter House*

Time and again, we hear that walking for 30 minutes a day—on most or all days of the week—provides significant health benefits. But walking in the wrong shoes, failing to wear reflective clothing at night or not taking a water bottle on a hot day will not only ruin your workout—it could lead to an injury. *Here's a quick guide to the best walking gear...**

WICK-ACTION SOCKS

Fitness walking should be done in athletic socks made of synthetic material, such as Cool-Max, Dri-Fit or Sorbtek, with cushioning in the heel and ball of the foot. These fabrics draw perspiration away from the skin to keep feet dry and prevent blisters.

Good brands: Asics, Thorlo, Nike, Wigwam. Wool socks from SmartWool are also good.

Typical cost: $6 to $15.

THE RIGHT SHOES

Good shoes are important. Expect to spend at least $65, and shop only in a store that specializes in athletic footwear. You can use a shoe made specifically for walking or a running

*These products are available at sporting-goods stores and at amazon.com. *All prices are approximate and subject to change.*

shoe with a low heel (which tends to be a little sturdier). Look for a shoe with a cushioned, flexible sole.

Shop at the end of the day, when your feet are largest. Wear your usual walking socks. If you use orthotic inserts, wear them as well. Before buying, walk around in the shoes for at least a few minutes inside the store. The heel should fit snugly, and there should be room to wiggle your toes.

Good brands: Any walking shoes made by Adidas, New Balance and Nike. But, if running shoes make more sense for you, consider Asics, New Balance and Saucony.

REFLECTIVE CLOTHING

Reflective clothing offers essential protection against cars—not only at night, but also when walking in the morning twilight or at dusk. The simplest solution is to wear a lightweight, reflective vest over your other clothes. Available in sporting-goods stores, bike shops and athletic-shoe stores, this type of vest starts at $15.

Good brands: Asics, Jogalite, Nathan and Nike.

Many sportswear manufacturers now offer sweat suits, shirts and shorts that have reflective strips.

WATER-BOTTLE CARRIER

Take along a water bottle so you can drink before, during and after your workout. You can buy clips, slings or waistpacks to carry your bottle. A bottle sling from Nathan costs $8.00.

PEDOMETER

When it comes to pedometers, the simpler the better. Fewer functions mean less chance of something breaking. A basic pedometer provides step count and distance walked.

Good models: The Sportline Distance/Safety Light Pedometer 348 will display the number of steps and the distance covered in miles or kilometers, with a built-in light ($25). Weighing just 0.75 ounce, Digiwalker SW-401 ($20) converts steps into miles, while the SW-701 ($30) will also calculate calories burned. Both come with security straps.

HEART-RATE MONITOR

Monitoring your heart rate can help you exercise more efficiently. It also helps people who are at risk for heart attack from pushing themselves too hard. Some basic heart-rate monitors are the Acumen and the Polar brands, each consisting of a lightweight chest-strap transmitter and a wristwatch-like display that registers your heart rate.

The Polar FS1 ($60) displays heart rate only. Acumen Eon Basix ES ($40) also comes in a smaller, women's version. Mio Heart Rate Monitor watches work without a chest strap. Instead, the wearer presses two fingers against a sensor to display heart rate and calories burned (starts at $35).

WALKING POLES

Lightweight aluminum and fiberglass poles—sold either as single walking staffs or as a pair of walking or trekking poles—allow you to push off with each step like a cross-country skier. This reduces strain on your knees and ankles while increasing the number of calories you burn.

The best single staffs are made by Tracks (*www.trackspoles.com*). These include the Lite Staff ($50), available in two lengths, with a weight of 10 to 11 ounces...the Sherlock Travel Staff for $90, providing adjustable length and a weight of 18 ounces, which unscrews for easier packing...and the Compact Travel Staff ($90), which weighs 10 ounces and collapses to 19 inches for storage.

When using two trekking poles, the proper technique is essential. Most poles come with instructions.

Good brands: Exel Nordic Walker Poles (starting at $70 per pair) are fiberglass walking poles with ergonomic grips. Exerstrider ($70 per pair) features a lightweight aluminum shaft with a durable rubber tip.

Emotional Healing

John W. James, founder of the Grief Recovery Institute in Sherman Oaks, CA, *www.grief-recovery.com*. He is the coauthor of *The Grief Recovery Handbook: The Action Program for Moving Beyond Death, Divorce and Other Losses*. HarperCollins.

The statement "Time heals all wounds" may be well-intentioned, but it does little to help a person who is grieving.

Time alone doesn't heal—it's what you do with the time that helps resolve the pain.

Everyone will experience loss from time to time—whether it's divorce, the end of a relationship or the death of a loved one. Although grief is a natural response to such events, we often deny the strong feelings.

Problem: Unresolved grief can result in depression and low energy levels. It can also weaken the immune system, which can lead to ulcers, the flu and other conditions.

Good news: By identifying and acknowledging the emotions associated with grief, you can learn to live with loss—rather than be consumed by it.

Here is how to help yourself—or a loved one—cope effectively...

HOW TO HELP OTHERS

After several days of sadness and emotional shock, the bereaved person inevitably begins to review his/her emotional relationship with the loved one. This is true with all losses, including divorce, job loss, the death of a loved one or even a beloved pet.

Relatives or friends of the griever can facilitate this process by listening in a nonjudgmental way and encouraging the person to talk about his feelings. *Here are several topics that a bereaved person needs to talk about...*

• **Circumstances leading up to the loss.** Grieving people have a strong need to explain exactly "what happened" in a safe setting, without having their reactions judged or being confronted with "insights" from the listener.

• **How the bereaved person found out about the loss.** Did he hear about it over the telephone? In person? Some other way? It's important to talk about how this news was relayed —and the emotions that accompanied it. This will help reduce the emotional tension attached to the bad news.

• **Stories about the loved one.** Hearing fond remembrances from other people helps put the relationship with the loved one into a much broader emotional context.

Even in the case of divorce, truthful memories are helpful. No one gets married anticipating a divorce.

HOW TO HELP YOURSELF

As the reality of loss sinks in, a grieving person also begins to think of things in the relationship that he might have done differently. *All* unresolved grief stems from these regrets. Following a loss, grievers wish they could turn back the clock and resolve these emotional issues. My research has shown that quite convincingly.

The following actions can be taken alone—or with the help of a partner who agrees to keep your conversations private...

• **Evaluate the relationship realistically.** There can be a tendency to enshrine someone who dies. Your loved one might have been a good person, but that does not mean he was perfect. In the case of a less-than-loved one or in a divorce, grievers may try to demonize the person.

An accurate memory of someone is always stronger and will be more cherished than a fantasy. Unless you remember your loved one as he actually was, it becomes impossible to complete your emotional relationship. Completion means you will be able to remember the relationship as it was without feeling devastating pain.

• **Create a time line of your relationship.** On a piece of paper, draw one horizontal line, representing the time you and your loved one spent together. The left end of the line is the beginning of your relationship.

Along this line, write significant junctures in your relationship. Record whatever comes to mind, along with the approximate date. If an event seems positive, write it above the line. List negative events below the line.

The time line will help you discover all the things that are unfinished. Although this may be difficult, it is essential to returning to a life that will have meaning and purpose.

• **Categorize your memories.** After you finish your time line, make a list of anything you wish you had done or said at these junctures. *Divide them into...*

• Amends (things that you feel the need to apologize for).

• Forgiveness (things you need to forgive the other person for).

• Other emotional statements. For example, "I love you" or "I appreciate the time you spent with me." Or, in the case of a less-than-loved one, "I hated the way you treated me."

• **Write a letter.** Now that you have identified all these undelivered messages, write a two-page letter to your loved one. It is best done by yourself, in a single one-hour session. *Example...*

"Dear Dad, I have been thinking a lot about our relationship, and I have discovered some things that I want to tell you..."

"Dad, I apologize for..." (Repeat this phrase for each undelivered amends on your list.)

"Dad, I forgive you for..." (Repeat this phrase for each item in your forgiveness category.)

"Dad, I want you to know..." (Repeat this phrase with each emotional statement on your list.)

When you're finished, be sure to conclude the letter with the word "good-bye" and the name of your loved one. *Example...*

"I love you and I miss you. Good-bye, Dad."

For best results, the letter must be read aloud to another person. In the case of divorce or estranged relationships, the letter must never be heard or read by the other person.

How to Be Happy... Yes, Happy!

The late Albert Ellis, PhD, a renowned psychologist as well as founder of The Albert Ellis Institute in New York City, *www.rebt.org*. He wrote more than 60 books, including *How to Make Yourself Happy and Remarkably Less Disturbable*. Impact Publishers.

When it comes to the pursuit of happiness, many people have it all wrong. They strive for a "perfect" life. If they can't boast of a sizable stock portfolio...a loving mate...and model children, they sink into despair.

The fact is, all of us have the power within us to make ourselves happy even in the face of severe adversity.

UNHAPPINESS vs. DISSATISFACTION

We all have personal goals—to succeed at work or at a sport...maintain loving relationships

31

...or master an art or hobby. If these goals are not met, we're certain to feel dissatisfied.

But we need not become depressed about it.

There is really nothing wrong with dissatisfaction. It spurs us on to improve our lives. The problem occurs when we become *defeated* by our dissatisfaction.

Sadly, this happens all too often, usually due to irrational and demanding beliefs.

FIRST STEP TO HAPPINESS

Identify the irrational belief that's behind this "must" thinking. Change it to an attitude of "I prefer." Preference has an implicit "but..."

Example: "I'd like to have an intimate partner, but it may take a long time to find one. In the meantime, I can be happy with my other relationships or even alone." This acknowledges the unpredictable and imperfect nature of our lives.

On the other hand, a demand is nonnegotiable. It leaves you with very little emotional leeway. If you don't get what you want, you become depressed or angry.

Example: "I must have a steady partner. If I don't find him/her, it proves that I am worthless."

This primitive thinking reflects the grandiosity of a child as he struggles to learn his limitations. Adults learn realism but may revert to grandiose thinking during periods of stress.

THE SECOND STEP

Try to develop a healthy attitude toward adversity. It's almost impossible to avoid. The trick is to learn to cope with obstacles without derailing your goals.

Important: Be willing to continually revise your goals.

Say that you have decided to play the violin only to discover that you have no aptitude for it. You can insist on playing your violin—and drive yourself crazy because you are not as good as you demand that you be. Or you can switch to the piano or another instrument that comes more naturally to you.

Exception: If you find a particular craft exceedingly difficult to master—but still within your grasp—you may want to persevere until you are proficient in it.

However, many people stick to unrealistic goals rather than look for more suitable alternatives. This is self-defeating.

It's similar to the lesson in Aesop's fable about the fox and the grapes. The fox wants the grapes but cannot reach them. When they prove unattainable, the fox derides them, saying they were probably sour anyway.

I say it is better to accept disappointment about the grapes, grab a banana instead—and move on!

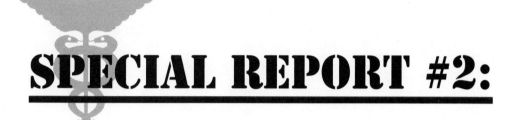

SPECIAL REPORT #2:

21st-Century
Health Breakthroughs

21st-Century Health Breakthroughs

Healthy Heart Prescription

Doctors have long believed that high blood cholesterol is the primary reason for the development of fatty plaque deposits in the arteries (atherosclerosis).

But research shows that a largely unrecognized cause of heart disease is actually blood viscosity. Or in other words, the thicker your blood, the greater your risk for clogged arteries.

If cholesterol really were to blame for atherosclerosis, *all* the body's arteries would be affected. In fact, heart patients tend to have plaque deposits only in the coronary arteries leading to the heart...the carotid arteries leading to the brain...and the femoral arteries that feed the leg muscles.

Why does this targeted buildup occur? Poor diet and an unhealthy lifestyle make the blood abnormally thick. This viscous blood creates friction along the arterial walls and forms plaque, much like a callus that forms on the hands.

How it works: Viscous blood forces the heart to pump harder, which elevates blood pressure. High blood pressure stretches the walls of the coronary, carotid and femoral arteries. These areas are particularly affected because of their proximity to the heart and the increased pressure that gravity exerts in the legs when standing. Exposed to the full force of the heart's pumping action, these areas gradually thicken and harden.

Hardened arteries increase blood pressure even more. This causes blood flow to become turbulent—the same way a smooth-flowing river turns into rapids as it heads through a narrow stretch. Over time, this process erodes the protective lining of your arteries.

Plaque deposits on the artery walls are actually the body's way of *repairing* this damage.

The late Kenneth R. Kensey, MD, a former research cardiologist at Michael Reese Hospital in Chicago, and coauthor of *The Blood Thinner Cure: A Revolutionary Seven-Step Lifestyle Plan for Stopping Heart Disease and Stroke.* Contemporary Books. He also was an inventor and founder of a company that developed new technologies for treating and preventing cardiovascular disease.

But if one of these deposits ruptures, it can trigger a heart attack or stroke by causing the artery to clog. Plaque also interferes with the flow of blood, causing buildup that can eventually lead to the artery's complete blockage.

CONTROLLING VISCOSITY

Blood viscosity is affected by the number of red blood cells you have...the flexibility of your red blood cells (each cell gradually stiffens over its 120-day life span)...and the thickness of your blood plasma (the liquid that surrounds your blood cells).

We don't yet have an approved technique for measuring blood viscosity. But a device I developed for this purpose, which simulates blood flow in the human artery, is now in clinical trials. In a few years, measuring your blood viscosity is likely to become as common—and important—as measuring your blood pressure is today.

HEART PROTECTION

Most people who are concerned about heart attack know to avoid tobacco, weight gain and high blood pressure.

Important: Hypertension is typically indicated by blood pressure of 140/90 or higher. But research shows that treatment should be considered for some patients whose blood pressure is above 120/80.

Treatment strategies include losing weight, eliminating sodium from your diet, restricting alcohol intake to two drinks per day and taking medication if necessary.

For even greater heart protection, ask your doctor about trying these simple strategies...

• **Donate blood.** Premenopausal women are at low risk for heart disease.

Reason: Their monthly menstrual flow lowers their red blood cell concentration and stimulates production of new, more flexible red blood cells—reducing the "sludge factor" significantly.

To replicate this blood loss, I recommend that men and postmenopausal women donate a pint of blood every eight weeks—the maximum permitted by the American Red Cross. According to a study conducted in Finland, men who donated blood were up to 10 times less likely to have a heart attack than the men who did not.

• **Forget the eight-glasses-a-day rule.** We are a dehydrated society.

Reason: We drink lots of caffeine, colas and alcohol, all of which rob the body of water. Even a slight water loss causes the blood plasma to thicken.

Water consumption lowers blood pressure and helps blood move through the arteries more easily.

I advocate consuming 12 eight-ounce glasses of water every day. If you get tired of water, try seltzer mixed with a little fruit juice.

• **Take aspirin.** Aspirin makes your blood platelets less sticky, which helps block the formation of plaque deposits.

One recent Harvard study found that taking aspirin daily cuts heart attack risk in half. I recommend taking 81 milligrams (mg) daily—the equivalent of one "baby aspirin."

Smart idea: To remember your daily aspirin, take the tablet every morning after you brush your teeth.

• **Take daily fish oil supplements.** Fish oil capsules contain the omega-3 fatty acids, which (unlike other varieties of fat) act as a "lubricant" in the bloodstream. This decreases blood viscosity.

We aren't sure why fish oil does this, but we do know that Eskimos, who regularly consume salmon and other fish rich in omega-3s, have almost no atherosclerosis.

To be sure you take fish oil daily, I recommend taking two 1,000-mg capsules every morning, right after your aspirin.

• **Do the *right* kind of exercise.** Thirty minutes of aerobic exercise, such as walking, jogging or biking, four days per week will strengthen your heart, lower your blood pressure and help you control your weight. It's important to drink one pint of water before starting exercise. Continue drinking throughout your workout—even if you don't feel thirsty.

Caution: Do *not* engage in exercise if you have uncontrolled high blood pressure. This will only accelerate the damage to your arteries.

• **Reduce psychological stress.** Most of us tend to downplay the role that stress can play in the development of heart disease. But the effects are not just theoretical. Research has shown that there are direct links between job stress and the progression of atherosclerosis. Stress raises blood pressure and hastens dehydration by increasing levels of the antidiuretic hormone, and this results in more frequent urination.

Heart patients who monitor stress utilizing biofeedback are 77% less likely to have a heart attack or require cardiac surgery, according to one recent study.

If you feel that stress is an issue in your life, ask your doctor to help you devise a stress-reduction program. This might encompass progressive muscle relaxation, breathing exercises, meditation, biofeedback-assisted relaxation, cognitive-behavioral therapy and/or stress-reducing prescription medication.

This Test Detects Heart Disease Earlier Than Ever Before

Heart disease can be detected early utilizing *electron beam computed tomography* (EBCT). This artery-scanning technique checks the heart for tiny calcium deposits, which are among the earliest signs of trouble.

In a recent study of women thought to be at modest risk for heart disease, EBCT found that many actually had the deposits. EBCT may be a good idea for women who are over age 50 and men over age 40, even if they do not have the known risk factors for heart disease, such as high triglycerides and/or LDL (bad) cholesterol and low HDL (good) cholesterol.

EBCT is a painless, five-minute test that can be performed in a hospital or an outpatient setting.

Lewis Kuller, MD, DrPH, professor of public health, former chairman, department of epidemiology, University of Pittsburgh Graduate School of Public Health.

Strategies for Controlling High Blood Pressure

Sheldon G. Sheps, MD, a cardiologist and emeritus professor of medicine at the Mayo Medical School in Rochester, MN. He is the editor of *Mayo Clinic on High Blood Pressure*. Mayo Clinic.

Most patients assume that high blood pressure (or hypertension) is relatively simple to diagnose and treat. Not so. Even experienced doctors can fail to effectively treat all the complexities of the condition.

To avoid many of the serious health threats associated with hypertension—heart attack, stroke, kidney failure, etc.—it helps to understand recent research findings...

• **Even mild hypertension needs treatment.** Optimal blood pressure is 115/75 or below. Traditionally, doctors have treated blood pressure only when readings climb to 140/90 or higher.

But research shows that a systolic reading (the top number) of 130 to 139 and a diastolic reading (the bottom number) of 85 to 89 can cause artery damage.* Blood pressure readings between 120/80 and 139/89 are defined as pre-hypertension.

Any increase in blood pressure needs to be lowered, either with lifestyle changes (a healthful diet, regular exercise, etc.) or medication.

• **Systolic pressure is just as important as diastolic pressure.** Many doctors continue to focus on diastolic pressure because they were taught it was the main cause of organ damage.

Fact: An elevated systolic pressure (140 to 150) needs to be lowered—even if your diastolic pressure is normal.

• **"Pulse pressure" may predict heart disease more accurately** than systolic and diastolic readings. Pulse pressure is the numerical difference between systolic and diastolic pressure. Some researchers now believe that pulse pressure is even more important than systolic pressure in determining long-term health risks.

*Systolic pressure is the force that is generated when the heart's main pumping chamber contracts. Diastolic pressure is that which occurs between these contractions.

A pulse pressure below 50 indicates that the arteries are elastic and healthy. But when arteries are stiff and inelastic, systolic pressure rises and diastolic pressure falls. This can increase pulse pressure to 60 or higher.

New medications: Vasopeptide inhibitors target pulse pressure by lowering systolic pressure while having relatively less effect on diastolic pressure. These drugs are not available in the US due to safety concerns. Currently there are no active clinical trials in the US.

• **Blood pressure readings taken in a doctor's office are not always enough.** People who regularly check their blood pressure at home control their hypertension more effectively than those who get only periodic readings in a doctor's office.

Bonus: Monitoring done in your home can detect two common types of faulty blood pressure readings...

• White-coat hypertension is a spike in blood pressure that occurs when people feel anxiety during a doctor's appointment.

• White-coat normotension is a drop in blood pressure that occurs in people who feel especially relaxed in their doctors' offices (compared with home or work).

Consider at-home monitoring if your blood pressure is mildly elevated during office visits ...or if you're being treated for high blood pressure. Your doctor can give you specific recommendations on the frequency. *For accurate home readings...*

• Use an electronic (digital) blood pressure-measuring device. Most models are easy to use. *Cost:* $30 to $400.*

Ask your doctor to measure your arm to determine the proper cuff size. Cuffs that are too small give artificially high readings. Cuffs that are too big give low readings.

• On the days you measure your blood pressure, take two readings during the morning (a few hours after you wake up)...and two in the evening ...then average the results. Always wait at least a half hour after eating...smoking...or drinking caffeine or alcohol to take your blood pressure.

*All prices subject to change.

Important: Go to the bathroom first. A full bladder tends to elevate readings.

• Bring a log of the readings to your next doctor's appointment. If the readings are unusually high—or are rising over time—call your doctor right away.

• **Salt really does matter.** New research shows that restricting salt intake to 1,500 milligrams (mg) daily—down from the current recommendation of 2,400 mg—can reduce systolic pressure by 11.5 points and diastolic pressure by an average of 5.5 points.

• **Drinking alcohol can raise blood pressure.** Excessive alcohol consumption is thought to contribute to hypertension in one out of 10 people who suffers from this condition.

Men should have fewer than two drinks per day...women, one.

• **Deep breathing helps.** People who practice deep breathing for 15 minutes daily—inhaling through the nose for approximately four seconds ...holding it momentarily...then exhaling through the mouth for four seconds—may reduce their blood pressure.

Helpful: The FDA has approved a prescription device called RESPeRATE for lowering high blood pressure. This device can measure breathing rate, then creates audio-guided exercises to slow down breathing.

More information: Contact the manufacturer, InterCure, at 877-988-9388 or on the Web at *www.resperate.com.*

• **Even minor weight loss makes a difference.** In one study, 40% of people with hypertension who lost eight to 10 pounds were able to stay off antihypertensive medication.

Key: Exercise regularly, eat less fat and cut your calories.

• **Exercise daily.** Most experts recommend exercising at least three days per week, but research shows that exercising every day or most days of the week can lower blood pressure by five to 10 points.

Best choices: Aerobic exercises, such as walking, biking or swimming.

Flu Vaccine Cuts Stroke Risk

Getting vaccinated against the flu cuts stroke risk in half—and even more in people who have been vaccinated for five consecutive years. The vaccine helps prevent influenza and resulting secondary infections, which cause inflammation. Inflammation is associated with atherosclerotic plaque buildup in the arteries. Rupture of this plaque leads to stroke.

However: The vaccine does not prevent stroke in those people aged 75 or older, maybe because high blood pressure and other conditions override this protective effect.

Self-defense: Talk to your doctor about receiving the flu shot every October.

Pierre Amarenco, MD, chairman of the Neurology and Stroke Center, Denis Diderot University, Paris. His study was published in *Stroke,* 1400 Western Rd., London, Ontario, Canada N6G 2V4.

An Integrated Approach To Rheumatoid Arthritis Is Much More Effective

Michael E. Weinblatt, MD, codirector, clinical rheumatology, Brigham and Women's Hospital in Boston. He is the author of *The Arthritis Action Program: An Integrated Plan of Traditional and Complementary Therapies.* Diane.

Two million Americans have rheumatoid arthritis (RA), a chronic and potentially disabling joint disease. RA is essentially the result of an immune system that has gone haywire.

Ordinarily, the antibodies and cells that comprise the immune system will protect the body against bacteria, viruses and other disease-causing invaders. But when things go awry, the immune system attacks the cartilage that lines the joints.

Result: Inflammation, swelling and pain... and eventually, destruction of cartilage and bone

In the last decade, researchers have developed a number of effective treatments for RA. These alleviate symptoms and, in most cases, slow the disease process—or halt it entirely.

FIRST LINE OF DEFENSE

Doctors used to postpone the use of "big-gun" RA drugs for as long as possible—to spare patients from side effects.

Now it's clear that RA can cause permanent disability within just a few years. Given this information, most physicians are opting to begin aggressive treatment within the first few months after diagnosis.

In many cases, the condition can be controlled with *ibuprofen* (Motrin, Advil, etc.), *naproxen* (Naprosyn, Aleve) or another nonsteroidal anti-inflammatory drug (NSAID).

NSAIDs reduce the pain and inflammation triggered by RA—but only when taken in dosages that are far higher than those used to treat headaches.

NSAIDs block inflammation-causing compounds called *prostaglandins.* Unfortunately, they also block a similar compound that protects the lining of the stomach.

That is why long-term use of high-dose NSAIDs often irritates the digestive tract.

As powerful as they are, NSAIDs do nothing to arrest the underlying disease process. For this, doctors rely on disease-modifying antirheumatic drugs (DMARDs). In most cases, a NSAID and a DMARD are prescribed together.

The relatively mild cases of RA are often treated with *hydroxychloroquine* (Plaquenil). This DMARD is often effective, but it can take six months to start working.

If hydroxychloroquine fails to control symptoms, doctors may also prescribe *methotrexate.*

Caution I: In rare cases, hydroxychloroquine can cause retinal damage. People taking the drug should see an ophthalmologist yearly.

Caution II: Methotrexate can cause liver damage in rare cases. Patients should undergo liver function testing every four to eight weeks while taking it.

Another DMARD, *sulfasalazine* (Azulfidine), is often prescribed alone for mild arthritis...or combined with methotrexate. These two drugs share many side effects.

THE NEWEST DRUGS

The most exciting news regarding treatment for RA is the emergence of *etanercept* (Enbrel) and *infliximab* (Remicade).

These so-called "biological response modifiers" are precisely targeted to block the action of *tumor necrosis factor* (TNF)—a compound responsible for much of the joint damage that is caused by RA.

Unfortunately, neither drug can be taken orally. Etanercept is injected twice a week (you can learn to do this at home). Infliximab is given intravenously every four to eight weeks.

These drugs are costly. One year's supply can cost more than $10,000.*

Some insurance plans cover these drugs, but they may also charge a 20% copayment.

COMPLEMENTARY APPROACHES

Many herbs, supplements, diets, etc., have been touted for relief from rheumatoid arthritis. Most lack scientific support, but there is some evidence that they can help reduce pain and inflammation.

Caution: Check with your doctor before taking any herbs or supplements—they may interfere with the effects of your prescription medication.

In addition, a physical therapist can prescribe exercises that may help relieve RA. An occupational therapist can help you perform daily activities correctly and can fit you with adaptive equipment, such as splints and a cane.

Ask your rheumatologist to give referrals to these specialists.

*All prices subject to change.

Delicious Soy Foods Help Beat Disease

Mark Messina, PhD, president of Nutrition Matters, Inc., and adjunct associate professor of nutrition at Loma Linda University School of Medicine in Loma Linda, CA. He is coauthor of *The Simple Soybean and Your Health*. Avery.

Why are soy foods becoming increasingly popular in the US? Besides their versatility and high nutritional value, these remarkable foods may protect against heart disease, osteoporosis and other serious health threats—especially cancer. Increasingly, research suggests that this is the case.

Tofu, tempeh, soy milk, etc., are all great sources of protein, calcium, folate, fiber and omega-3 fatty acids.

What makes soy foods even more special is their high content of the *isoflavones*. These chemical compounds imitate the salutary effects of estrogen.

Isoflavones also help to neutralize the free radicals—harmful oxygen molecules that are believed to contribute to a variety of serious health conditions.

Consuming one or more daily servings of soy foods may reduce the risk for two common types of cancer...

•**Prostate cancer.** An isoflavone called *genistein* appears to inhibit the growth of prostate cancer cells.

Example: Genistein may block the conversion of testosterone into a more potent compound called dihydrotestosterone, which fuels prostate tumors.

Studies involving thousands of men have shown that one daily serving of soy is associated with as much as a 70% reduction in the incidence of prostate cancer.

In the absence of clinical studies, of course, we can't be certain that soy *prevents* prostate cancer. But even a delay in tumor development would have a significant impact on the health of men.

•**Breast cancer.** Rats fed a soy-based diet are 25% to 50% less likely than other rats to develop breast cancer.

Human studies have yielded mixed results. When researchers compared women who had breast cancer to healthy women, they found little difference in soy consumption.

Another study found, however, that girls who consume 1½ servings of soy every day between ages 13 and 15 are 50% less likely to develop breast cancer later in life. Eating soy foods early in life may be particularly protective against breast cancer.

Theory: Isoflavones may make breast cells differentiate into mature cells earlier in life, so that they are less likely to undergo cancerous changes.

Important: Some breast tumors are stimulated by estrogen—and these could, in theory, respond similarly to the soy isoflavones. Any woman who has been diagnosed with "estrogen-sensitive" breast cancer should discuss soy consumption with her physician.

ADDING SOY TO YOUR DIET

To gain soy's health benefits, aim for 50 milligrams (mg) of isoflavones and about 10 to 15 grams (g) of soy protein daily.

A wide range of foods now contain soy. *Some popular choices...*

• **Tofu** (a smooth, fermented product with a bland taste). One-half cup contains about 30 mg of isoflavones and 10 to 12 g of protein.

• **Tempeh** (chunky, tender soybean cake). One-half cup contains approximately 60 mg of isoflavones and 16 g of protein.

• **Soy milk.** One cup contains about 25 mg of isoflavones and 7 g of protein.

• **Miso.** One cup contains about 80 mg of isoflavones and 30 g of protein.

• **Soy nuts.** One-half cup contains approximately 170 mg of isoflavones as well as 25 g of protein.

Other sources of soy: Breakfast cereals, energy bars, soy pastas and soy-milk beverages.

Textured vegetable protein, a low-fat meat substitute made from soy, can be used in casseroles, sauces, hamburgers, etc.

Whole soybeans are also a good choice because they're rich in isoflavones, protein and fiber.

Bonus: Whole soybeans, along with soy milk, contain *oligosaccharide* sugars that nourish "friendly" bacteria in the colon, which may reduce the risk for colon cancer.

SOY SUPPLEMENTS

Health-food stores sell dozens of soy supplements in pill form. Each pill typically contains 25 to 50 mg of isoflavones.

Don't take them if your goal is to lower cholesterol. It's the protein in soy—which isn't found in these supplements—that does the job.

If you want isoflavones—*and* soy protein—opt for powdered supplements. However, further study on the effects of soy supplements is needed. Consult your health-care provider before staring a regimen of soy supplements.

Important Breakthroughs In Cancer Care

The late Gerald P. Murphy, MD, former director of research at the Pacific Northwest Cancer Foundation and Northwest Hospital, both in Seattle and former chief medical officer of the American Cancer Society. He was also coauthor of *Informed Decisions: The Complete Book of Cancer Diagnosis, Treatment and Recovery.* American Cancer Society.

National Cancer Institute. *www.cancer.gov.*

Have cancer researchers found a cure for cancer? That tantalizing possibility was raised by a *New York Times* article that described an experimental therapy developed by Dr. Judah Folkman, a researcher at Children's Hospital in Boston.

Dr. Folkman had cured cancer in lab mice using the experimental drugs *endostatin* and *angiostatin,* also known as angiogenesis inhibitors.

Since Dr. Folkman's work, a number of angiogenesis inhibitors for cancer treatment have been discovered. The US Food and Drug Administration (FDA) has approved *bevacizumab* (Avastin) for use with other drugs to treat colorectal cancer that has spread to other parts of the body. Other angiogenesis inhibitors are currently being tested in clinical trials.

Good news: Antiangiogenesis therapy is just one of several recent breakthroughs in cancer therapy. *Many of the other breakthroughs are available right now...*

CONFORMAL RADIATION

With conventional radiation therapy, physicians know only the position of the tumor they are bombarding with radiation.

Since they don't know the tumor's shape, it's hard for them to limit the delivery of radiation only to the cancerous tissue. Some radiation inevitably "spills over" onto healthy tissue.

With conformal radiation therapy, doctors use three-dimensional imaging technology to plot the shape and position of the tumor. That way, high doses of radiation can be delivered accurately and with minimal damage to the surrounding healthy tissue.

GAMMA KNIFE

Used to treat brain tumors, this noninvasive tool can focus radiation with surgical precision.

The gamma knife is less risky than conventional surgery or radiation therapy. Brain tumors can be removed with little or no damage to surrounding tissue.

Recovery time is faster, too. In most cases, the treatment lasts less than one hour and the patient goes home the next day.

Conventional brain surgery typically requires at least three days in the hospital and four to six weeks of at-home recovery. Approximately 125 cancer centers in the US are now equipped with a gamma knife.

LYMPHATIC MAPPING

With cancers that spread through the lymphatic system—such as cancer of the breast and melanoma—surgeons used to remove not only the cancerous organ but also most or all of the lymph nodes under the armpit. This can lead to *lymphedema,* a painful and disfiguring swelling of the arm. It can also leave the arm highly vulnerable to infection.

A procedure known as lymphatic mapping helps prevent lymphedema by limiting the number of lymph nodes removed. After the tumor is cut out—while the patient is still on the operating table—dye is injected near the tumor site. By noting where the dye drains into the lymphatic system, the surgeon can pinpoint which lymph nodes should be removed and examined for cancer. That permits less extensive surgery.

RADIOACTIVE SEEDING

In conventional radiation therapy, radiation from a machine is beamed at the tumor. But researchers have found that radiation can be delivered more effectively to certain tumors by seeding them with tiny radioactive pellets.

The pellets deliver radiation to cancerous tissue without damaging nearby healthy cells.

Known as *brachytherapy,* this seeding technique has proven effective for cancers of the prostate and pancreas.

Used against prostate cancer, brachytherapy has proven just as effective as conventional radiation therapy and surgery—with a smaller risk for impotence or incontinence.

MONOCLONAL ANTIBODIES

Chemotherapy is often highly effective at killing cancer cells. But since the drugs used in chemotherapy affect healthy cells as well as cancerous ones, patients undergoing chemotherapy often experience toxic reactions, such as impaired heart, liver or kidney function.

Using gene-splicing technology, researchers cloned cancer-killing antibodies directly from the cells of cancer patients. These monoclonal antibody drugs attack cancer cells—but leave healthy cells alone.

The first monoclonal antibody drug to hit the market, *rituximab* (Rituxan), was approved by the FDA, and has proven highly effective against non-Hodgkin's lymphoma and rheumatoid arthritis.

FINDING GOOD CANCER CARE

With so many new cancer treatments now available, how can cancer patients be sure that they're receiving state-of-the-art care?

One way is to be treated at a facility funded by the National Cancer Institute (NCI).

The NCI funds more than 60 cancer centers in the US. To find out if there's one near you, contact the NCI at 800-422-6237 or *www.cancer.gov*. You can also call this number to learn about treatment options and clinical trials.

First-rate cancer care is also available at institutions accredited by the American College of Surgeons (ACS).

About 1,500 cancer facilities have the ACS accreditation. To find an accredited facility near you, check the ACS Web site at *www.facs.org* or call them at 800-621-4111.

Breast Cancer Breakthrough

New technology spots breast tumors $1/100$ the size of the smallest that can be seen with mammography or magnetic resonance imaging (MRI). During a *routine operative breast endoscopy* (ROBE), a viewing scope (or endoscope) about the thickness of a pencil lead is threaded into the nipple. Breast tissue appears 60 times normal size. Physicians can identify tumors early enough to increase the odds that the woman can undergo minimally invasive surgery. ROBE is especially useful for women with nipple discharge. It is available in many hospitals across the US.

William Dooley, MD, professor of surgical oncology, University of Oklahoma School of Medicine, Oklahoma City.

restaurants or other settings where they are exposed to secondhand smoke.

Kimberly Yolton, PhD, research associate, General and Community Pediatrics Research, Cincinnati Children's Hospital Medical Center.

Better Prostate Cancer Detection

During the typical prostate biopsy, six samples of suspicious cells are taken. However, this technique misses up to one in seven prostate malignancies.

Recent research suggests that taking 10 to 12 cell samples can uncover 14% more cancers. Taking additional samples results in higher lab fees, but this technique could save money and worry in the long run by eliminating the need for follow-up biopsies.

If you're scheduled to undergo a prostate biopsy: Ask your doctor about testing more samples.

Robert Bahnson, MD, professor, division of urology, Ohio State University Medical Center, located in Columbus.

Cholesterol-Lowering Medications May Stop Alzheimer's

Certain cholesterol-lowering drugs may also help to prevent Alzheimer's disease and other dementias.

Recent finding: Patients prescribed any of the class of drugs known as *statins* were 37% to 70% less likely to develop dementia than were similar people not taking a statin. Although the statins are widely used for preventing heart disease and stroke, further research is still needed before they can be recommended for dementia.

David A. Drachman, MD, professor and former chairman, department of neurology, University of Massachusetts Medical School, Worcester.

Secondhand Smoke May Lower Children's Intelligence

Passive smoking is already known to cause respiratory and behavior problems in kids.

In one study involving more than 4,000 children between the ages of six to 16, the higher a child's blood levels of *cotinine*, a by-product of nicotine, the worse he/she performed on intelligence tests. One parent smoking even less than a pack a day could raise a child's blood levels enough to reduce intelligence quotient (IQ) by about two points.

Self-defense: Parents should stop smoking. Also, do not take children to cigarette smoke–filled

Helpful Treatments for Macular Degeneration

Robert D'Amato, MD, PhD, director, Center for Macular Degeneration Research, Children's Hospital Boston. He is the coauthor of *Macular Degeneration: The Latest Scientific Discoveries and Treatments for Preserving Your Sight.* Walker & Company.

Until recently, there was no way to prevent age-related macular degeneration (AMD) or halt the disease's gradual—but persistent—deterioration of the eye's light-sensitive retina.

AMD affects one in three Americans over the age of 65. In its mildest form, the condition results in blurred vision and difficulty reading. But it can quickly progress to a more advanced form that causes blindness.

The disorder affects the *macula,* the region of the retina that is responsible for "central vision."

43

This enables us to read, recognize faces, drive and perform other activities that require sharp vision.

Most cases of macular degeneration begin with the formation of *drusen*—small yellow deposits that develop just behind the macula. Known as "dry" AMD, this condition can persist for years, generally causing only minor vision problems.

Unfortunately, one in 10 of those who are diagnosed with dry AMD go on to develop "wet" AMD. This form occurs when blood vessels under the retina leak fluid and form scar tissue, damaging or distorting the smooth surface of the retina. Wet AMD can rob a person of central vision.

Good news: Recent research confirms that a healthful diet and prudent lifestyle choices can reduce your risk of developing AMD. Moreover, a number of treatments are highly effective at minimizing vision loss in the early stages of the disorder.

Other treatments will reduce the blood vessel damage associated with wet AMD. *These include…*

• **Laser therapy,** an effective way to help stop the progression of AMD. During the 30-minute outpatient procedure, a high-powered laser seals off the leaky blood vessel.

Laser therapy is recommended if the blood vessel is clearly visible and located to the side of the retina. This allows the ophthalmologist to control any vision loss that can result from tissue damage caused by the laser therapy.

• **Photodynamic therapy** (PDT), a promising new form of laser therapy that uses a photo-sensitive dye, is available at many teaching hospitals. It causes less tissue damage than traditional laser therapy. For this reason, PDT is the preferred treatment. However, it must be repeated every few months.

Clinical trials are also being held to determine the effectiveness of other new treatments…

• **Submacular surgery** removes the blood vessel through a hole in the side of the retina. This procedure is being tested on patients whose damaged blood vessel is located in the center of the retina, which diminishes the success of laser surgery.

• **Transpupillary thermotherapy** uses a low-temperature laser, which limits damage to the retina and surrounding tissue.

• **Radiation therapy** uses a beam of electromagnetic energy to destroy the leaky blood vessels in much the same way that radiation is used to treat cancer. However, results from current trials have not shown a large benefit from radiation therapy.

• **Antiangiogenesis drugs** block the proteins that are critical to the formation of blood vessels that lead to AMD.

More information on clinical trials: Contact the National Eye Institute, 301-496-5248, *www.nei.nih.gov.*

Safe Remedy for Ringing in the Ears

Seventy percent of those with ringing in the ears got at least partial relief from an injection of the common anesthetic *lidocaine,* according to one study. The injection was given in the middle ear and in the arm on three consecutive days.

Good news: The lidocaine therapy, given along with the antianxiety drug *alprazolam* (Xanax), was effective against both high-tone tinnitus (ringing, hissing, whistling, ticking) and low-tone tinnitus (roaring, buzzing, popping or swishing). The quieting effect seems to be permanent—but the treatment can be safely repeated, if necessary.

John J. Shea, Jr., MD, chief otologic surgeon, Shea Ear Clinic, Memphis.

All About Prolotherapy

Jan Guthrie, founder and director of the medical information and research company, The Health Resource, 933 Faulkner St., Conway, AR 72034.

Robert G. Klein, MD, an internist and prolotherapist in private practice in Santa Barbara, CA.

Chronic back pain, whiplash injuries to the neck and many other types of musculoskeletal pain that are not helped by physical therapy, painkilling medication or chiropractic manipulation can often be controlled via *prolotherapy*.

In this highly effective but little-known treatment, small amounts of an irritant solution—usually concentrated glucose—are injected into the painful area.

The resulting inflammation promotes growth of collagen, the protein that's a major component of ligaments, the cable-like structures that hold our joints together.

New collagen growth helps reduce pain and increases joint stability by strengthening the fibrous capsule around joints. It also brings significant improvement in joint mobility.

Many forms of chronic musculoskeletal pain are caused by ligament damage. Car accidents, falls or repetitive movements cause ligaments to loosen and/or tear. Prolotherapy is effective for most ligament-related pain.

SIDE EFFECTS

Prolotherapy patients generally feel fine for four to eight hours after the injections because a local anesthetic is given along with the irritant. Any discomfort that follows should slowly subside over the next several days.

Many individuals who undergo prolotherapy experience pain, swelling, soreness, temporary stiffness and bruising at the injection site. Fortunately, discomfort can usually be minimized by medication, ice and massage.

Caution: Smoking makes the therapy less effective, as does the use of aspirin and other anti-inflammatory drugs.

PRECISION COUNTS

Most patients need a series of injections over a period of several weeks or months. In some cases, prolotherapy is teamed with other forms of soft-tissue treatment—such as physical therapy, joint manipulation or acupuncture.

Prolotherapy injections must be given *precisely* at the junction of a bone and a ligament. Misplaced injections are ineffective and possibly dangerous. If the irritant is inadvertently injected into the spinal canal, for instance, paralysis or even death could occur.

Consequently, prolotherapy injections must be administered only by a clinician thoroughly trained in the technique. Some say that orthopedic surgeons are ideal for administering prolotherapy injections. That is because they have a thorough knowledge of the location of ligaments and muscles.

FINDING A PROLOTHERAPIST

Only about 300 orthopedic physicians and osteopaths in the US and Canada currently use prolotherapy in their practices.

Among these practitioners is former Surgeon General C. Everett Koop, MD. He began using prolotherapy in the early 1960s, after another doctor used it on him to cure the once-intractable pain in his neck and arm.

For more information about prolotherapy, contact the American Association of Orthopaedic Medicine at *www.aaomed.org*. There is limited quality data supporting the use of prolotherapy. More randomized controlled trials are needed.

INSURANCE COVERAGE

One prolotherapy session costs about $90 to $300.* The number of treatments required depends upon both the severity of the pain and the patient's response to the treatment.

Some major health insurance organizations cover prolotherapy. Others decline coverage because they consider it to be an "unproven" or "experimental" treatment.

*All prices subject to change.

Better Hip Surgery

A recent hip fracture surgery causes less blood loss and requires a shorter hospital stay than conventional hip surgery. *Percutaneous compression plating* involves implanting two screws through two one-inch incisions. Developed in Israel becoming widespread in the US, the procedure stabilizes the hip and minimizes further bone damage, even in patients with osteoporosis. Most patients can stand up almost immediately after surgery. The procedure is available at several medical centers throughout the US.

Robert D'Ambrosia, MD, professor and chairman of orthopedic surgery, University of Colorado, Denver.

The Ultimate Age-Defying Diet

Bradley J. Willcox, MD, principal investigator of geriatrics, Pacific Health Institute, Honolulu, HI, and assistant professor of geriatrics, University of Hawaii. He is co-principal investigator of the Okinawa Centenarian Study and coauthor, with his twin brother, D. Craig Willcox, PhD, of *The Okinawa Program: How the World's Longest-Lived People Achieve Everlasting Health—and How You Can Too.* Three Rivers Press.

For years, US government scientists have been urging Americans to consume at least *five* daily servings of fruits and vegetables. But that's not nearly enough, according to new research.

For maximum longevity, a better approach can be found in the fruit- and vegetable-rich diet of the world's longest-lived people, the men and women of Okinawa, Japan.

During 25 years of study, researchers have found that Okinawans have healthier arteries… lower risk for hormone-dependent malignancies, such as breast and prostate cancer…stronger bones…sharper minds…lean, fit bodies…and excellent emotional health.

Okinawans eat mainly high-carbohydrate, low-calorie, plant-based foods—the same diet deemed optimal for long-term health by more than 2,000 scientific studies.

At first glance, the Okinawa diet seems like a lot of food to eat each day. The trick is to remember that a daily serving, as defined by the US Department of Agriculture (USDA), is actually quite small.

Examples: For raw, leafy vegetables, a serving is one cup. For whole grains, a serving is one-half cup of cooked cereal, one slice of bread or half a bagel.

When you follow the Okinawa program, in which plant-based foods comprise two-thirds of the diet, you'll exceed USDA dietary recommendations.

Here's how scientists have adapted the Okinawa diet for Americans…

• **Eat until you are 80% full.** Okinawans say, *hara hachi bu:* "Eat until you are eight parts full" (out of 10).

Restricting calories is a proven way to prolong life and vitality. By eating fewer calories, your body will create fewer free radicals—the molecules responsible for the biochemical damage that causes aging.

This does not mean Okinawans eat *less*. In fact, they eat more food by weight than most North Americans. But it's important to note that Okinawans eat small amounts of fat and sugar, which are calorie-dense.

To eliminate excess calories…

• Flavor meals with spices instead of fat.

• When cooking, spray the oil instead of pouring—two seconds of spraying equals one-half teaspoon of oil.

• Start your lunch with a chunky, low-fat soup. If you do, you'll eat 20% fewer calories.

• When dining out, order lean fish instead of steak…ask for fatty sauces and dressings to be served on the side…and share desserts.

• **Eat nine to 17 servings of vegetables and fruits daily.** A diet rich in fruits and vegetables decreases your risk for heart disease, cancer, stroke, high blood pressure and obesity.

Fruits and vegetables are full of healthful nutrients—but low in calories. They also contain antioxidants, which help to protect you against free radicals.

To boost your intake of fruits and vegetables…

• For breakfast, eat a fruit salad that contains cantaloupe, strawberries, blueberries and apples.

• At lunch, include vegetables like tomato, broccoli and celery in your salad.

• At dinner, make vegetable soup that includes onion, zucchini and carrots.

• **Eat seven to 13 servings of whole-grain foods daily.** Whole grains are rich in nutrients, antioxidants and fiber. These important parts of your diet decrease your risk for many illnesses, including heart disease, stroke, diabetes and cancer.

Many different types of whole grains—from amaranth, barley and bulgur to rice, triticale (a high-protein hybrid of wheat and rye) and wheat—can be found in cereals, breads and pastas.

For maximum benefit: Choose breakfast cereals that contain at least 7 grams of fiber per serving.

•**Eat two to four servings of calcium foods daily.** Calcium fights osteoporosis and may help prevent colon cancer, high blood pressure and premenstrual syndrome. Good plant sources of calcium include green, leafy vegetables…calcium-fortified soy products, such as tofu and soy milk…and calcium-fortified orange juice.

Important: Low-fat dairy products may *not* be the best source of calcium. The protein in dairy products can leach calcium from your bones.

•**Eat two to four servings of flavonoid-rich foods daily.** Blood levels of flavonoids—beneficial compounds found in all plants—are up to 50 times higher in the Japanese than in white Americans, according to a new study. A high-flavonoid diet may help prevent heart disease as well as breast, prostate and colon cancers.

Isoflavone-rich soy products contain flavonoid levels that are up to 1,000 times greater than those found in other foods.

Flaxseed contains high amounts of lignans, which are similar compounds. Beans are another good source, followed by tea, onions and apples.

To increase your intake of flavonoids and lignans…

•Eat soy products twice a day. Choices include tofu, miso (a salty paste often used as a flavoring), soy milk, soy nuts and soy burgers.

•Take one tablespoon of flaxseed oil daily, or use it instead of butter or as a salad dressing.

•Drink three cups of black or green tea each day.

•Emphasize flavonoid-rich fruits and vegetables, such as broccoli, kale, celery, onions, snow peas, turnip greens, apples, strawberries, grapes and apricots.

•**Eat one to three servings of omega-3 foods per day.** Most Americans do not get enough of the omega-3 fatty acids. These dietary constituents protect your brain, arteries and immune system.

To boost your intake of omega-3 foods…

•Eat fatty fish (salmon, tuna or mackerel) three times a week.

•Add flaxseed to your diet. Mix it into cereal or pancake or muffin batter.

•Avoid red meat. It may increase your risk for colon and prostate cancer. If you must eat red meat, limit it to no more than three times a week—and choose lean cuts.

•**Drink fresh water.** You need adequate hydration. But forget about the eight-glasses-a-day rule. Drink enough so that your urine is clear.

Do Apples Fight Baldness?

Procyanidin B-2, a compound in apples, has been found to increase the number and thickness of hair shafts—in just six months.

However: The compound was applied topically, so it is not known whether eating apples will have the same benefit. Until more research is completed, consider eating four apples with the skin a day or take a supplement containing procyanidin.

Tsukuba Research Laboratories, Ibaraki, Japan.

Nobel Prize Winner's Breakthrough—Prevent Heart Attack and Stroke With Nitric Oxide

Louis J. Ignarro, PhD, corecipient of the 1998 Nobel Prize in Medicine for his research on nitric oxide. He is also a professor of molecular biology at the University of California, Los Angeles, School of Medicine, and the author of *No More Heart Disease.* St. Martin's.

One small molecule produced by the body may do more than any drug to prevent heart attack and stroke.

Nitric oxide, a gas that occurs naturally in the body, is critical for healthy circulation. It helps dilate blood vessels, prevent blood clots and regulate blood pressure, and it may inhibit the accumulation of arterial plaque.

HOW IT WORKS

Nitric oxide is a signaling molecule primarily produced by the cells in the endothelium (inner lining) of blood vessels. A signaling molecule fits into docking sites (receptors) on cell walls and triggers biochemical reactions. *Nitric oxide helps prevent heart disease and stroke by...*

• **Expanding blood vessels.** Nitric oxide protects the blood vessels' smooth muscle tissue from harmful constriction, and this allows blood to circulate with less force. Some doctors report that elevating nitric oxide in hypertensive patients can lower blood pressure by 10 to 60 points.

• **Controlling platelet function.** Platelets, cell-like structures in blood that can clump up together, may form blood-blocking clots, the main cause of heart attack and stroke. A vascular network that is enhanced by nitric oxide sheds platelets and inhibits dangerous clots.

• **Reducing arterial plaque by 50%.** Arterial plaque, which consists of fatty deposits in the coronary arteries, is the underlying cause of heart disease. Nitric oxide is an antioxidant that inhibits the passage of monocytes, a type of immune cell, into the artery wall. This in turn reduces the underlying inflammation that promotes plaque.

• **Lowering total cholesterol by 10% to 20%.** That's a modest decrease—but there's some evidence that nitric oxide is even more effective when combined with the cholesterol-lowering statins. Nitric oxide lowers cholesterol through its antioxidant properties. The preliminary research suggests that stimulating nitric oxide production in people who have elevated cholesterol makes it possible to lower their statin doses by at least 50%.

TO BOOST NITRIC OXIDE LEVELS

It is not yet known how much nitric oxide normally is present in the body or what levels are optimal. This gas is difficult to measure because it disappears almost instantly upon exposure to air. Research scientists can measure levels with electrodes inserted in blood vessels. Simpler tests are needed before doctors can measure nitric oxide as part of standard checkups.

Beginning in early adulthood, nitric oxide levels gradually decline, probably due to damage to the endothelial cells caused by such factors as a high-fat diet and a sedentary lifestyle.

Nitric oxide can't be taken in supplement form because it's a gas. However, patients can take other supplements that increase production of nitric oxide in the blood vessels. *These supplements, all available at health-food stores, have few if any side effects...*

• **L-arginine,** an amino acid found in meats, grains and fish, passes through the intestine into the blood. From the blood, it enters endothelial cells, where it is used to make nitric oxide.

A Mayo Clinic study found that people taking L-arginine showed significant improvement in endothelial function and blood flow compared with those taking placebos. It is hard to get sufficient L-arginine from food, so supplements are recommended.

Dose: 2,000 to 3,000 milligrams (mg) taken twice daily—for a total of 4,000 to 6,000 mg.

• **L-citrulline.** Supplemental arginine doesn't enter cells readily unless it is combined with L-citrulline, another amino acid. Melons and cucumbers are rich sources of L-citrulline, but they don't provide high enough levels to significantly increase nitric oxide levels.

Dose: 400 to 600 mg daily.

• **Daily multivitamin that includes vitamin E.** Vitamin E helps reduce the assault of cell-damaging free radicals on the endothelial lining and may promote higher levels of nitric oxide. The amount of vitamin E that is in most multivitamin/mineral supplements is about 50 international units (IU), an effective dose.

Warning: Don't take the high-dose vitamin E supplements. Recent studies suggest that people who take daily doses of 400 IU or higher may be more susceptible to heart disease and other illnesses.

• **Vitamin C.** Like vitamin E, vitamin C will decrease oxidation in the blood vessels and may cause an increase in nitric oxide. People who consume high levels of vitamin C experience a reduction in arterial plaque, which is associated with higher levels of nitric oxide. You can get vitamin C from food, but I recommend supplements because they are so convenient and easy to take.

Dose: 500 mg daily.

DIET AND EXERCISE

In addition to taking supplements, it is important to maintain a healthy lifestyle by watching what you eat and being active. *Try to...*

•**Do aerobic exercise for at least 20 minutes three days a week.** It stimulates endothelial cells to continuously produce nitric oxide, even on days that you don't exercise.

•**Minimize intake of saturated fat.** Saturated fat, found in such animal products as red meat, poultry, butter and whole milk, contributes to the accumulation of arterial plaque and impairs nitric oxide production.

Better: Olive oil, fish and flaxseed. The fats found in these foods help protect the endothelium by elevating levels of beneficial HDL cholesterol and lowering the harmful LDL form.

•**Consume more fiber.** The dietary fiber in grains, fruits and vegetables lowers blood pressure and LDL cholesterol and raises HDL, thereby protecting endothelial cells.

Bonus: Many of the foods that contain fiber are also rich in antioxidants, which inhibit the cell damage that lowers nitric oxide. Eat at least 25 grams of fiber daily—and drink at least eight eight-ounce glasses of water each day to make sure that the fiber moves through your system properly.

•**One hour before bedtime,** take a hot bath scented with lavender oil.

•**After your bath,** drink warm milk with honey.

•**Go to bed by 10:30 p.m.**

Ayurveda teaches that our biological rhythms make the hours of sleep which occur before midnight the most rejuvenating.

Deepak Chopra, MD, founder of the Chopra Center for Well Being in Carlsbad, CA, and a foremost leader in integrative medicine. Dr. Chopra has written numerous books on health, including *Grow Younger, Live Longer.* Three Rivers Press.

Singing Silences Snoring

Studies have found that even those people who cannot carry a tune snored less after performing vocal exercises 20 minutes a day for three months.

Theory: Singing tones up the flabby throat muscles that cause snoring.

If you snore: Before trying singing, ask your doctor about sleep apnea. This potentially dangerous airway disorder causes sufferers to stop breathing repeatedly during the night. Sleep apnea may require surgery or another type of treatment.

Edzard Ernst, MD, PhD, director of the department of complementary medicine, Peninsula Medical School, Exeter, England.

For a Better Night's Sleep...

Humans need eight hours of sleep every night. *My recommendations...*

•**Eat a light dinner** no later than 7 p.m.

•**Take a short, leisurely walk** after dinner.

•**After 8:30 p.m.,** minimize mentally intensive activities, such as paperwork.

Turn Off Your Fat Genes For Lasting Weight Loss

Neal Barnard, MD, president of the Physicians Committee for Responsible Medicine in Washington, DC, *www.pcrm.org.* Dr. Barnard is the author of *Turn Off the Fat Genes—The Revolutionary Guide to Taking Charge of the Genes That Control Your Weight.* Harmony Books.

The findings of the Human Genome Project have helped scientists to uncover crucial facts about our genetic makeup—

including the genes that control our weight. Although some genes, such as those for eye color, have a fixed outcome, our weight genes simply *suggest* certain tendencies.

Good news: If you learn to work with the genes that affect your sense of taste, appetite and other eating habits, you'll be amazed at how easily you can shed unwanted pounds.

Six key strategies…

KNOW YOUR TASTE GENES

One out of four people is a "super taster." They taste flavors more acutely—especially bitter foods like broccoli or grapefruit. Another one out of four people has a blunted sense of taste and doesn't mind bitter flavors. The rest of us fall somewhere in the middle.

To determine how your sense of taste influences your eating habits, ask yourself: Do you dislike cabbage? Brussels sprouts? Does grapefruit juice seem intolerably bitter? Is coffee impossible to drink without milk or cream? Do sugary desserts or snacks taste sickeningly sweet?

If you answered "yes" to three or more of these questions, you're probably a super taster. Although you're unlikely to overeat or indulge in sweets, you may avoid vegetables that are essential for optimum health.

Solution: Eat sweeter vegetables, including carrots, sweet potatoes and green beans. When eating "unpleasant-tasting" vegetables, be sure to cook them for a few extra minutes to reduce their bitterness. Serving them with a sour topping, such as lemon juice or a vinegar-based dressing, also will help to counteract their bitter taste.

If you answered "no" to at least three of the questions, you probably have no aversion to eating greens—but you run the risk of shoveling in large quantities of food without thinking, especially fatty snack foods.

Solution: Choose low-fat foods, such as bananas, apples and any vegetable or whole-grain food, so that you can afford to eat larger quantities.

GET ENOUGH CALORIES

One of the key genes for controlling your weight—located on chromosome #7—manufactures a hormone called *leptin,* which influences your appetite. When the leptin levels decline, you feel hunger.

A low-calorie diet reduces leptin levels. For example, a 1,000-calorie-a-day diet cuts leptin levels in half.

Result: An appetite "rebound" that makes you hungrier than ever. Reducing calories will also slow the rate at which your body burns off calories during your diet—and for several weeks afterward.

Make sure you get enough calories to maintain your leptin level—no fewer than 1,400 calories per day is recommended.

BOOST YOUR METABOLISM

Some people are born with a naturally fast metabolism, in which their bodies burn calories rapidly. Others have a slower metabolism.

The foods you consume also influence your metabolism. Foods rich in complex carbohydrates maximize "after-meal burn" (the number of calories you expend while digesting food) for several hours after eating.

To increase your after-meal burn, eat more legumes (beans, peas and lentils)…fruits, such as apples, bananas, oranges and pears…green vegetables, such as asparagus, broccoli and spinach …sweet potatoes…and whole grains, such as brown rice, barley, whole wheat, pumpernickel or rye bread and oatmeal.

These foods also tend to be high in fiber, so they empty from your stomach at a slow and steady rate. This helps control your appetite.

AVOID DIETARY FAT

Several popular diets blame carbohydrates for weight gain. But studies have shown that body fat comes almost exclusively from dietary fat—thanks to one gene on chromosome #8, which produces an enzyme called *lipoprotein lipase* (LPL).

Located in the capillaries running through your body's fatty deposits and your muscles, LPL converts dietary fat into a form your body can use—either storing it as body fat or burning it for energy.

A high-fat diet not only gives this enzyme more raw material to work with, but it also boosts the level of insulin in your blood. That, in turn, increases the amount of "fat-storing" LPL in the fat cells, while decreasing the amount of "fat burning" LPL in your muscles.

To minimize fat-storing LPL, you must cut way down on dietary fat—including animal *and* vegetable fat.

What's the most effective way to do this? Switch to a vegetarian diet that contains no meat or dairy products. This so-called "vegan" diet also curbs your intake of vegetable oils. For more information on vegan diets, contact the Vegetarian Resource Group, 410-366-8343, *www.vrg.org*.

GIVE DIETARY CHANGES TIME

Cutting down on fatty foods may seem hard at first. That is because your taste buds have become accustomed to their daily "fix" of fat. Your taste buds do have a memory, but it lasts only three weeks.

If you do give up a particular food for three weeks, your craving for it will significantly decline. It's important not to cheat. Even one slip will reactivate your craving.

AIM FOR GRADUAL WEIGHT LOSS

The healthiest way to lose weight is at a rate of about one pound per week. If you follow all the eating suggestions outlined above, you should be able to reach this goal.

Weight-Loss Tip

To cut back on food intake, consume several small meals during the day instead of three large ones...or eat from a smaller plate so that it appears you have more food.

Put your fork down after every bite. This will encourage you to eat more slowly, giving your stomach time to signal that you are full.

The late Robert N. Butler, MD, professor of geriatrics at Mount Sinai School of Medicine and president of the International Longevity Center, both in New York City. In 1976, Dr. Butler won a Pulitzer Prize for his book *Why Survive? Being Old in America.* Johns Hopkins University Press.

Better Than Stretching

Stretching before exercise may *not* reduce the risk for injury. Although fitness experts have long recommended stretching to limber up the muscles before exercise, a recent review of studies shows there is no strong evidence to support this advice.

Better warm-up: Perform the activity you're preparing to do at a lower intensity for 10 minutes or until you break a sweat.

Examples: Walk before jogging...hit a tennis ball against a wall before playing tennis...run some dribbling drills before playing basketball.

Ian Shrier, MD, PhD, past president, Canadian Academy of Sport Medicine, Gloucester, Ontario.

The Myth About Sit-Ups

Peggy W. Brill, PT, a board-certified clinical specialist in orthopedic physical therapy with a private practice in New York City. She is coauthor of *The Core Program—15 Minutes a Day That Can Change Your Life.* Bantam Books.

There is a myth that sit-ups and crunches are excellent forms of exercise. In fact, the *worst* thing you can do is force yourself to do sit-ups or abdominal crunches. These exercises push your head out of alignment and cause tension in the shoulders.

Although sit-ups and crunches strengthen the *rectus abdominus* (the muscle that runs from the pelvis to the rib cage), they tend to elongate the *transverse abdominus* (girdle) muscle, causing the lower abdominals to pouch. In addition, sit-ups and crunches can damage the spine.

To work *all* the muscles of your abdomen in the most effective way possible, try this safe and easy exercise...

•**Dead bugs.** Lie on your back with knees bent and head and feet flat on the floor. Tuck in your chin to elongate your neck, then cough to contract your oblique muscles and to pull the rib cage down and in.

Next, holding the abdominal contraction as tightly as you possibly can, lift your arms high above you toward the ceiling. Extend one arm up over your head and the other arm toward your feet. Then reverse the motion. Alternate arms for a count of 30.

Keeping your abdomen contracted and your chin tucked in, extend your arms toward the ceiling and lift both knees toward your chest. Make a gentle bicycling motion with your knees for a count of 30.

Finally, combine the arm and leg movements and do both at once. When one leg moves toward your chest, the arm on that same side should reach over your head. Continue for a count of 60.

Make sure to keep your abdomen contracted and your lower back pressed into the floor throughout the exercise. An arch in your back can cause back strain.

The exercises here can be performed in 10 minutes, once a day. A padded exercise mat is all you need to get started.

Illustrations by Shawn Banner.

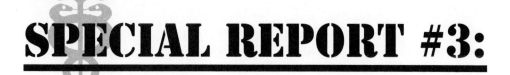

SPECIAL REPORT #3:

How to Beat
Health Care
Dangers and Rip-Offs

How to Beat Health Care Dangers and Rip-Offs

Does Your Doctor Give The Ultimate Checkup?

The managed-care revolution has drastically reduced the amount of time doctors are able to spend with their patients. During the typical office visit, your doctor barely has time to investigate troublesome symptoms and check your weight...pulse...heartbeat...blood pressure, etc. That is just not enough.

A thorough exam should also address your overall physical and emotional well-being diet ...lifestyle...and any "silent" symptoms that can increase your risk for health problems.

Most doctors take a medical history, listing current health problems...prescribed medications ...allergies, etc. This information is critical.

Helpful: When writing down your concerns, give your doctor additional information that he/she may fail to include in the medical history...

- **How's your diet?**

- **Are you taking any herbal or dietary supplements?**

- **Do you get enough sleep?**

- **Are you physically active?**

- **Are you experiencing sexual problems?**

Also mention if you smoke, how much alcohol you drink and whether you're having difficulty in your personal relationships. Try to keep the list to one page.

THE PHYSICAL

To save time, doctors often take shortcuts during the physical. This can affect not only your current diagnosis and treatment—but also your future health. *Here are steps that are most commonly omitted...*

- **Blood pressure.** This vital sign is typically checked in one arm while the patient is sitting. For a more accurate reading, blood pressure

Leo Galland, MD, director, Foundation for Integrated Medicine, which promotes a comprehensive approach to health care, New York City. He is author of *The Fat Resistance Diet*. Broadway. *www.fatresistancediet.com.* Dr. Galland is a recipient of the Linus Pauling award.

should be tested in *both* arms, preferably while you're lying down.

If blood pressure differs by 15% or more between arms, there may be blockages in the large blood vessels.

Important: If you're taking blood pressure medication—or if you get dizzy when you change positions—your doctor should check your blood pressure immediately after you stand up. If blood pressure drops by more than 10%, a change in dosage of blood pressure medication may be needed.

•**Eyes.** Most people visit an ophthalmologist or optometrist. But if you don't see an eye specialist regularly and you're age 40 or older, your internist or family practitioner should measure the pressure on your eyeballs to test for glaucoma and look for lack of lens clarity—an early sign of cataracts.

Bonus: A careful eye exam can also reveal blood vessel narrowing or small hemorrhages on the retina—indicators of vascular conditions that increase your heart disease risk.

•**Hamstrings.** Few doctors test these muscles at the back of the thighs to identify potential back problems. To do so, the doctor should ask you to lie on your back and lift each leg to a 90° angle.

If you can't perform the lift, you may need a stretching program to relax the hamstrings.

•**Lymph nodes.** The lymph nodes in your neck are typically checked, but doctors should also check those in the groin and under your arms. Swollen lymph nodes may signal infection. Lumps could indicate cancer.

•**Pulse points.** Your doctor probably checks your pulse in your neck and/or groin—but may skip your feet. If pulse strength differs in these three areas, it can be a sign of peripheral arterial disease.

•**Skin.** Many doctors ignore the skin altogether, assuming that it should be examined by a dermatologist. Not true. The skin should also be checked during a general medical checkup.

To examine your skin, your doctor should ask you to disrobe so he can look for moles on every part of your body, even your scalp and the bottoms of your feet.

If you have moles larger than one-half inch—or if your moles have gotten larger, darkened or changed their shape—you should get a referral to a dermatologist for a melanoma screening.

•**Thyroid.** This butterfly-shaped gland at the base of the neck is often missed during the lymph node exam. By palpating the thyroid, your doctor can screen for thyroid cancer.

FOR WOMEN ONLY

•**Breasts and reproductive organs.** Most doctors check the breasts for suspicious lumps, but few doctors show women how to perform monthly exams at home.

Helpful: When performing a self-exam, move all eight fingers, minus the thumbs, up and down instead of in a circle. That way, you will be covering the entire breast.

If you don't see your gynecologist regularly, your physician should also perform rectal and vaginal exams. These exams should be performed simultaneously—it makes it easier to identify suspicious masses.

FOR MEN ONLY

•**Testicles and rectum.** When examining men who are age 40 or older, most physicians do perform a digital rectal exam to screen for prostate cancer. However, they often neglect to perform a testicular exam to check for testicular cancer. Your doctor should also teach you how to perform a testicular self-exam.

Beginning at age 50—even earlier if there's a family history of prostate cancer—every man should undergo a prostate-specific antigen (PSA) blood test, performed every three years...or more often if abnormalities are found.

LABORATORY TESTS

Routine blood tests include cholesterol levels ...liver and kidney function...blood glucose levels ...and a white blood cell count. But other blood tests can be important if a patient shows signs of certain conditions. *These blood tests include...*

•**C-reactive protein.** An elevated level of this inflammation marker can indicate heart disease risk.

•**Homocysteine.** An elevated level of this amino acid is associated with heart disease and stroke risk.

Helpful: The B vitamin folate, when taken at a dosage of 200 to 400 micrograms daily, reduces homocysteine levels.

- **Iron.** A genetic condition or excess dietary intake of this mineral can cause iron overload (*hemochromatosis*).

- **Lipoprotein (a).** Elevated levels of this blood protein increase the risk for blood clots.

- **Magnesium.** Low levels of this mineral can bring about fatigue, generalized pain and/or muscle spasms.

- **Zinc.** If you are deficient in this immune-strengthening mineral, you may be prone to frequent infection.

How to Choose a Primary Care Doctor

After choosing an HMO primary-care doctor, set up a "get-acquainted" appointment. If you have a chronic ailment, ask how much experience he/she has in treating it, and how readily he/she will refer you to a specialist.

Remember: Do not ignore your instincts—if you don't have confidence in a doctor when you're healthy, odds are you won't like him when you're sick either. Most HMOs will pay for the appointment.

Alan Steinberg, MD, an internist in private practice in Marina del Rey, CA. Dr. Steinberg is the author of *The Insider's Guide to HMOs*. Plume.

How to Find a Good Naturopathic Physician

Jamison Starbuck, ND, a naturopathic physician in family practice in Missoula, Montana. She is a past president of the American Association of Naturopathic Physicians and a contributing editor to *The Alternative Advisor: The Complete Guide to Natural Therapies and Alternative Treatments*. Time Life.

Naturopathic physicians (or NDs) have practiced medicine in the US since the 1890s. But most people do not know how to find an ND or how to add such a doctor to their health-care team.

NDs perform the same basic duties as family physicians, and NDs treat everything from colic to cancer. Patients select NDs instead of medical doctors when they want nutritional advice and natural medicine, including homeopathy and botanical medicine, in lieu of prescription medication and surgery.

Several US states,* plus Puerto Rico and the Virgin Islands, currently license NDs. In these areas, NDs practice as primary-care physicians, specializing in natural medicine. NDs diagnose and treat disease, perform physical exams, refer patients to specialists, prescribe both natural and certain pharmaceutical medicines, do physical therapy and minor surgery.

If your state does license NDs, contact your attorney general's office for the phone number of the board that oversees NDs. They can give you information on the scope of practice and a list of licensed doctors.

If you live in a state that does not license NDs, search the Yellow Pages under "Physicians, Naturopathic," or ask a health-care professional you trust to recommend an ND. Be aware that in unregulated states, practitioners with little or no training may call themselves "naturopaths." Before your appointment, ask the ND you have selected about his/her academic training, clinical experience and license to practice.

The American Association of Naturopathic Physicians (AANP) is a good source for finding a qualified ND. Members of the AANP must be graduates of a naturopathic medical college and/or hold a state license to practice naturopathic medicine. Go to the AANP's Web site, *www.naturopathic.org,* for a list of physicians by state. You can also call the AANP toll-free at 866-538-2267 to get more information.

If you want to work with both a traditional medical doctor and an ND, make sure each practitioner is willing to share information about you—diagnoses, changes in medication, etc. A cooperative team approach is your best bet in achieving optimum health.

*States that license NDs are Alaska, Arizona, California, Connecticut, District of Columbia, Hawaii, Idaho, Kansas, Maine, Minnesota, Montana, New Hampshire, North Dakota, Oregon, Utah, Vermont and Washington.

Get the Respect You Deserve in the Hospital

Charles B. Inlander, a consumer advocate and health-care consultant based in Fogelsville, Pennsylvania. He was founding president of People's Medical Society, a consumer health advocacy group active in the 1980s and 1990s. He is the author of more than 20 books, including *Take This Book to the Hospital with You.* St. Martin's.

A hospital stay should be a time of healing. But all too often the experience erodes a patient's personal dignity.

Here's how to ensure that your needs are met during hospitalization...

•**Ask about *everything*.** Let your doctors and nurses know that you plan to play a major role in your care. Inquire about your treatments and prognosis.

Don't worry that your doctor will think you lack confidence in him or her. Or that asking questions will cause resentment among the hospital staff, producing worse care.

Studies have shown that hospital patients who ask questions receive better and more respectful treatment. Questions encourage the medical staff to pay more attention to you.

If hospital personnel use medical jargon, ask them to explain it.

Always inquire about the medication you are given. If you receive a new drug, ask, *Why is this different from what I was getting before? Who ordered it?*

Asking questions also helps prevent medical mistakes. Nearly 100,000 hospital patients die every year from medical errors, such as wrong medications and botched surgery.

•**Know who is treating you.** Hospital staffing levels have been drastically reduced. A person in a white uniform is not necessarily a doctor or nurse. In fact, it may be someone with almost no training, such as an orderly.

If someone comes into your room to perform a procedure—and you don't know who that person is—ask, *Who are you? What do you do here?*

If you are concerned that the person is not fully trained in the procedure, refuse it. You'll be surprised at how quickly you receive treatment from a nurse.

•**Don't be shy about seeking help.** If no one responds to your call button within a few minutes, pick up the phone. Call the hospital operator and ask to be connected to the nursing station on your floor.

When the phone is answered, say you need help in your room—immediately.

Important: If you have a complaint, you have the right to a response in a reasonable period of time. If you're not getting one, ask to see the hospital's "patient representative" or "ombudsman," who mediates between staff and patients. See what the representative can do to resolve your situation.

If there is no patient representative or the representative is not helpful, ask to see the medical director or the hospital administrator.

•**Have someone with you at all times.** If you are seriously ill or undergoing surgery, you probably won't have the energy or mobility to protect your rights. So have someone with you 24 hours a day.

Enlist family and friends, and work out a schedule. As long as your "advocate" is not interfering with the delivery of care, he has a right to be there.

•**Talk to the staff about a schedule that fits your needs.** A shift change may be the only reason a nurse is taking your blood pressure at midnight. If that's the case, tell your doctor or the head nurse that you'd prefer not to be awakened at night.

•**Make sure the food is appetizing.** Notify the hospital dietitian if fresh fruits and vegetables aren't served...the food doesn't arrive prepared at the proper temperature...the meals are served at unusual times for the convenience of the staff... or you lack sufficient time to eat.

Better: If your doctor permits it, have visitors bring food to supplement hospital meals. Make sure they are aware of any special dietary restrictions you have.

•**Know your rights.** You have a right to say *no* to any medical procedure. You have the right to see your medical records. You have the right to check yourself out at any time, even against the advice of hospital personnel. You have the right to fire your doctor. You have the right not to be treated by a medical student, if you so choose.

What Hospitals Don't Want You to Know

Timothy McCall, MD, a board-certified internist in Oakland, California, medical editor of *Yoga Journal* and author of *Yoga As Medicine.* Bantam. Dr. McCall leads workshops and retreats on yoga and yoga therapy around the country and worldwide.

Hospitals are fighting for survival. Cutbacks from the federal government and from managed-care plans have reduced their revenue streams. Throughout the US, hospitals are closing, merging or implementing draconian cost-cutting measures.

But it's not just hospitals that are at risk. Corner-cutting also threatens the well-being of patients. *Here's what hospitals don't want to tell you—and what you can do about it…*

• **They're discharging patients "quicker and sicker."** To save money, hospitals are routinely discharging patients much earlier than they used to. If they plan to send you home, be sure you'll have the support services you may need, such as visiting nurses and physical therapists, and that family members will be able to perform any duties expected of them. If you do not feel your condition or home circumstances make discharge safe, alert your physician. If necessary, file an appeal with your insurer.

• **They've cut their nursing staffs.** Even though doctors get most of the glory, it's the nurses who run hospitals. They monitor your condition, administer medications and make sure medical equipment functions properly. But maintaining a skilled nursing staff is expensive, so hospitals have found it cheaper to substitute "aides," many of whom have very little bedside training.

You have the right to inquire about the qualifications of anyone who will treat you. Ideally, your primary nurse will be a registered nurse (RN). It's best if each nurse working on a typical medical or surgical ward is caring for no more than five patients or no more than two in an intensive-care unit.

If the nurse-to-patient ratio is higher than that, consider having family members stay with you while you're hospitalized or, if you can afford it, hire a private-duty nurse.

• **They reuse disposable medical equipment.** Some medical equipment—such as a dialysis catheter that is intended for single-use—is cleaned and reused, raising concerns about infection and product failure. Although reusing equipment is not illegal, you should ask that only new equipment be used.

• **They do not report inferior doctors.** Although the law mandates that incompetence or any misconduct among physicians must be reported to the federal government, 60% of all hospitals have never filed even a single disciplinary report in the last decade. Part of the reason is that doctors are hospitals' "cash cows." They have the power to direct their patients to competing hospitals, so there's an incentive to not make waves.

Your best bet: Avoid potentially dangerous doctors by learning as much as you can about your condition and the medications used to treat it. The more you know, the better your ability to spot a bad apple.

• **They overwork residents and interns.** Although current regulations do cap the work hours of doctors-in-training, these limits may be routinely violated. If you are admitted to a teaching hospital, ask your resident or intern how many consecutive hours he has been working. Thirty-six-hour shifts are still routine. If you are concerned, it's your right to refuse care from anyone who looks too exhausted to provide it.

If you believe a hospital is doing anything that imperils patients, I recommend reporting it to your state's regulatory authority or contacting the not-for-profit Joint Commission on Accreditation of Healthcare Organizations at 800-994-6610 or *www.jointcommission.org.* Their e-mail address is *complaint@jointcommission.org.*

More from Dr. Timothy McCall…

PSA Testing: More Harm Than Good?

One of the most common questions I get from my male patients is whether they should have the *prostate-specific antigen* (PSA) test. This simple blood test, I tell them, can detect prostate cancer at a very early stage. What isn't known is whether getting a PSA test will benefit *you*.

In 2011, there were approximately 240,000 newly diagnosed cases of prostate cancer in the US. It causes more than 30,000 deaths every year, and is now the second leading cause of cancer death in American men (lung cancer is the leading cause of death).

Prostate cancer is very common. It has been estimated that 40% of all men over the age of 50 have it. But only about 8% of men ever demonstrate symptoms, and only 3% die of the disease. In other words, four out of five men with prostate cancer never have symptoms, and nine out of 10 will die of something else. In the past, most of these men never even knew they had prostate cancer.

The PSA test changed all that. Before the test went into widespread use—beginning in the mid-1980s—there were only about one-third as many cases diagnosed per year. Even so, the number of prostate cancer deaths was about the same as it is today.

This points out one of the biggest problems with PSA testing. We now have the ability to detect cancer not just in those destined to die of the disease but also in the majority who will never get symptoms. Unfortunately, it is impossible to differentiate between the two groups—at least so far.

The second big problem with PSA testing is that it's not clear that the standard treatments for prostate cancer—radical prostate surgery and X-ray therapy—save lives. Many doctors and patients assume that they do. But no good studies have ever demonstrated their effectiveness. Such studies are now under way, but the results won't be available for several years. In the meantime, the number of men undergoing prostate surgery has skyrocketed.

The side effects of radical prostate surgery, such as impotence and incontinence, are significant. Although surgeons working at the top prostate cancer centers report better results, a survey taken two to four years after the operation found that only 11% of men had had an erection sufficient for intercourse in the prior month. Almost a third required adult diapers or clamps on their penises to help control their

urine. Radiation therapy also has significant side effects.

There are major disagreements among medical authorities about PSA testing. The American Cancer Society says men should have one every year starting at age 50 (earlier if they're African-American or have a family history of prostate cancer). The US Preventive Services Task Force does not recommend routine screening.

For my male patients over age 70 and for those whose life expectancy (because of other illnesses) is less than 10 years, I advise against PSA tests. The side effects of treatment simply outweigh the benefits. I tell younger men that a PSA test could save their lives—or it could cause them a lot of needless grief. Right now, no one can tell you which.

I encourage my patients to learn as much as possible about prostate cancer. Visit your local library or go on-line. But remember, information more than a couple of years old is outdated. One Web site, OncoLink (*www.oncolink.com*), is a great place to start.

Given the uncertainties, whether to have the PSA test is a highly personal decision—one each man must make in consultation with his doctor. As with any medical decision that hinges mostly on value judgments, however, it should be *your* values—not your doctor's—that dictate what you do.

How to Avoid Unnecessary Surgery

Eric A. Rose, MD, former surgeon-in-chief and chairman of the department of surgery at the Columbia University College of Physicians and Surgeons in New York City. He is the author of *Second Opinion: The Columbia Presbyterian Guide to Surgery.* St. Martin's Press.

Few patients get all the facts they need to make prudent choices about surgery. Busy, intimidating doctors often gloss over important details about a proposed operation ...or overwhelm you with information—much of it beyond the comprehension of the average patient.

If your doctor recommends surgery: Learn the risks of the operation…how it should help you…and whether nonsurgical alternatives are an option. If the surgery will cause significant risk or discomfort, get a second opinion. *Be especially cautious if you've been advised to have surgery for…*

BACK PAIN

Severe back pain results when one or more discs—the tough, doughnut-shaped "cushions" that support the spinal vertebrae—degenerate or tear. This causes the disc to press against nerves, triggering intense back or leg pain.

Back surgery (discectomy) to remove the damaged portion of a disc will often provide relief—but not always. The potential benefit must be weighed against the risk for infection or, in rare cases, paralysis.

Doctors are often too quick to recommend back surgery. If you're having your first episode of back or leg pain, you probably don't need an operation. Symptoms often improve—without treatment—in six to eight months.

Surgery is strongly advisable only in patients who experience severe chronic pain or suffer pressure on a spinal nerve, causing paralysis or loss of bowel or bladder control.

CARPAL TUNNEL SYNDROME

People who often perform repetitive hand motions (such as typing) will sometimes develop chronic pain in their wrists and hands.

If the pain is chronic and severe, carpal tunnel release surgery is usually a good idea. In this 30- to 60-minute outpatient operation, the surgeon cuts the ligament to relieve nerve pressure.

Unfortunately, many surgeons recommend the surgery even for mild to moderate pain. In these cases, the pain can almost always be controlled with a wrist splint and/or physical therapy.

GALLBLADDER DISEASE

As long as gallstones aren't causing significant symptoms, they can be safely left in place.

But it makes sense to remove gallstones if an acute infection develops—or if abdominal pain occurs, especially after eating fatty meals. What's the best way to remove stones? *Laparoscopic cholecystectomy.* In this procedure, the surgeon creates four small incisions through which surgical instruments and a small viewing scope are inserted.

The scar tissue from previous surgeries can make laparoscopic cholecystectomy impractical. These cases require *open cholecystectomy.* This one- to three-hour procedure involves a five-inch abdominal incision and a three- to 10-day hospital stay.

HEART DISEASE

Coronary artery bypass graft (CABG) surgery restores blood flow to the heart when one or more coronary arteries are blocked. During this operation, a blood vessel harvested from the chest or leg is sewn on the affected artery on either side of the blockage, "bypassing" the damaged area.

This popular procedure is major surgery. It carries the risk for infection and postsurgical complications, such as pneumonia and stroke.

Heart bypass surgery can be a lifesaver if the blockage includes the left main coronary artery. Without the operation, such a patient has a 30% chance of dying within three years. People who have multiple blockages—especially ones near the heart—also benefit from this procedure.

But not all cardiac problems require bypass surgery. Even some seemingly severe cases can be treated with balloon angioplasty. During this less-invasive procedure, a catheter with a balloon attached is inserted and inflated to clear the obstructed coronary artery.

In certain cases, many people do fine without surgery. Nitroglycerine pills can be used to increase blood flow and aspirin can reduce blood clots. Beta-blockers, such as *propranolol* (Inderal) or *nadolol* (Corgard), can also be beneficial.

PEPTIC ULCER

Today, surgery for peptic ulcer (partial gastrectomy and vagotomy) is rarely recommended. That's because medications control the production of stomach acid so effectively. These medications include over-the-counter H_2-blockers, such as *cimetidine* (Tagamet) and *ranitidine* (Zantac)

...and prescription proton-pump inhibitors, such as *omeprazole* (Prilosec) and *lansoprazole* (Prevacid).

Bleeding ulcers usually do require surgery. However, the preferred operation is a minimally invasive endoscopic procedure. During this technique, a small, lighted viewing scope that introduces the surgical instruments is inserted through the mouth and into the stomach or small intestine.

PROSTATE CANCER

Prostate cancer that grows rapidly is life-threatening. For these cases, removal of the prostate gland (prostatectomy), radiation treatments and/or hormone therapy may be necessary.

But many prostate tumors grow so slowly that they are unlikely to cause any long-term problems. Some doctors do recommend surgery for these cases.

But "watchful waiting" may be a more reasonable alternative. Instead of operating, the doctor monitors the tumor using CT scans... and the patient watches for symptoms, such as difficulty urinating or urinary infections. Only then does surgery or other treatments become necessary.

What Surgeons May Not Tell About Joint Surgery

Ronald Grelsamer, MD, chief of patello-femoral reconstruction in orthopaedics at Mount Sinai School of Medicine in New York City. He is the author of *What Your Doctor May Not Tell You About Knee Pain and Surgery*. Warner Books.

Each year, thousands of Americans have their chronically arthritic hips or knees removed and replaced with prosthetic devices made of metal and plastic.

Ninety-five percent of these prostheses are still working effectively 10 years later, studies have shown.

However, complications can occur. These include infection, blood clotting, loosening of the prosthesis or persistent pain. *Here's what*

you need to know before undergoing a joint replacement...

• **Not all orthopedic surgeons are equally qualified to perform hip and knee replacement.** In recent years, the orthopedics field has grown tremendously. There are now thousands of orthopedic surgeons, but only a fraction of these surgeons focus their practice on hip and knee replacement.

If you're considering a hip or knee replacement, ask your family physician to refer you to an orthopedist who specializes in joint replacement of the hip and knee.

For a list of orthopedic surgeons in your area, contact the American Academy of Orthopaedic Surgeons, 847-823-7186, *www.aaos.org*.

• **There is no such thing as "urgent" hip or knee replacement surgery.** If a doctor tells you that a painfully arthritic joint "must be taken care of right away"—beware.

In an arthritic knee or hip, the smooth cartilage coating the joint's surface gradually wears away, until bone starts grinding against bone.

This condition may be painful, but it never requires emergency surgery. Arthritis pain waxes and wanes. Most episodes of acute pain subside after a few days or weeks.

Because the joint implants tend to wear out over time, I urge my patients to hold off on this operation for as long as possible. The patient should tell the doctor when he is ready for joint replacement surgery—never the other way around.

Consider an implant if the pain becomes too frequent and severe to control with medication. This gives the patient plenty of time to carefully sort through all the options.

• **Many doctors are too quick to perform multiple imaging tests.** X-rays are typically used to detect arthritic damage in the joint. If an X-ray indicates such damage *and* you have intractable pain, hip or knee replacement is usually warranted.

Some doctors routinely order magnetic resonance imaging (MRI) scans to check for torn cartilage. However, this is almost always a waste of time and money. Torn cartilage is irrelevant in the face of arthritis.

●**It's easy to pick the wrong prosthesis.** There are many prosthetic implants on the market. Ask your doctor about the track record of the particular prosthesis you're considering.

If you are over age 55: A tried-and-true prosthesis is usually preferable.

All hip and knee implants tend to loosen over time. By choosing a proven prosthesis, you reduce your chances of needing a second surgery later in life to replace the implant. As people age, this is especially important because replacement surgery is associated with a higher risk for complications.

Some older models last 20 years or longer. Many new models do not hold up as well as the best of established implants—but it typically takes years to discover this. An inferior model might wear out in a few years.

If you're under age 55: Newer implants and techniques may offer benefits. An increasing number of younger people are electing to have hip replacement—generally because of damage from a hip fracture or avascular necrosis (death of tissue in the hip).

However, doctors have not yet developed a fully satisfactory total joint-replacement technique for people of this age. As a result, these patients almost always require at least one additional surgery to replace the implants that have become loose and/or infected.

For this reason, younger patients should consider all available options, particularly the popular "cementless" technique that allows the bone to grow and fuse with the implant, instead of using cement to hold it in place. When choosing this type of implant, ask your surgeon for a model that has been used successfully for at least 10 years.

●**Dental problems can be dangerous for people with joint implants.** Bacteria can easily travel through your bloodstream from your mouth to your artificial joint, where it can cause infection. If possible, avoid dental work for one year after a joint-replacement operation.

Alert your dentist about your hip or knee prostheses. Make sure that he gives you an oral antibiotic before and after any dental surgery. Gum infection, bladder infection and ingrown toenails also pose an infection risk to your artificial joint. Such infections should be treated immediately.

How to Get the Best Emergency Care

Rebecca Shannonhouse, editor, *Bottom Line/Health,* 281 Tresser Blvd., Stamford, CT 06901.

Recently, I accompanied my friend—who was in excruciating pain—to a crowded emergency room (ER). After nearly *four hours* of waiting, she was diagnosed with kidney stones and given a painkiller.

This is no rare occurrence. As the demands placed on ERs increase, it is more important than ever to know the shortcuts to top-quality emergency medical care. To learn about these steps, I spoke with Gideon Bosker, MD, editor in chief of *Emergency Medicine Reports. His advice is outlined below...*

●**Respond quickly.** If you are over age 65 or you have a chronic condition—such as diabetes, heart disease or cancer—and experience a sudden change in your health, call 911. If an ambulance transports you to the ER, you should receive immediate care.

●**Get your doctor involved.** If possible, call your doctor *before* the ambulance arrives. He will notify the ER that you are on the way. This ensures that a physician will give you prompt attention. If you are not sure whether to go to an ER, call your doctor for advice. Don't hesitate to use his emergency number—page him, if necessary.

●**Take an escort.** It helps to have an advocate in the ER to act as a "constructive nag." Your friend can help describe your symptoms in order of severity.

●**Bring your medications.** This information helps the ER physician to make informed decisions.

Better: Carry an up-to-date list of your medications—and your doctor's contact information—in your wallet.

•**Wear a MedicAlert bracelet.** These special medical ID tags alert medical technicians and physicians to allergies or health problems, such as a heart condition, Alzheimer's disease or a history of stroke. To purchase one, call 888-633-4298 or visit *www.medicalert.org.*

Medical Red Flags: When to Go to the Emergency Room

Marie Savard, MD, an internationally recognized internal medicine physician, expert on wellness and champion for patient rights. She is the author of *How to Save Your Own Life.* Grand Central. Her Web site is *www.drsavard.com.*

Most of us know to see a doctor if we detect a suspicious lump or changes in a mole. If severe chest pain occurs, even a stoic will head to the nearest emergency room.

Other symptoms are easier to miss—or *dismiss.* But prompt diagnosis and treatment will protect your health...and possibly save your life—or that of a loved one.

Here are several red flags that may signal a medical emergency...

ABDOMINAL DISTRESS

Persistent cramps, bloating, vomiting or a change in appetite or bowel habits can indicate a variety of problems.

Best-case scenario: Spastic colon...viral infection...lactose intolerance...or indigestion.

Worst-case scenario: An ulcer...tumor ruptured appendix...ovarian cyst...intestinal obstruction...inflammatory bowel disease...or inflammation of the digestive tract, gallbladder or pancreas.

Seek emergency treatment: If you're vomiting and have not moved your bowels or passed gas in 24 hours—or if you have sudden, acute abdominal pain accompanied by fever—you may require emergency surgery.

Note: If your condition is serious enough to warrant emergency treatment, it's probably best

to avoid driving. Call 911 or ask someone to take you to the nearest hospital.

For milder discomfort, eliminate possible culprits, including aspirin, caffeine, alcohol, dairy products and artificial sweeteners. Try easing any symptoms with an over-the-counter product, like Maalox or Pepto-Bismol.

See your doctor: If symptoms persist for one week, get a checkup.

COUGH

A dry, nonproductive cough that lasts for more than two weeks requires medical attention.

Best-case scenario: Post-nasal drip...acid reflux...or continuing irritation from coughing.

Worst-case scenario: Infection...severe asthma...lung cancer...malignancy of the lymphatic system (known as lymphoma)...or congestive heart failure.

See your doctor: Get a physical exam and chest X-ray within one week.

HEADACHE

The worst headache of your life—especially if accompanied by vomiting—should not be ignored.

Best-case scenario: Acute viral infection ... or migraine.

Worst-case scenario: A leaking aneurysm ...infection of the lining covering the brain and spinal cord (bacterial meningitis), when accompanied by fever and stiff neck...or brain tumor.

Seek emergency treatment: You will need to undergo a CT scan or magnetic resonance imaging (MRI) scan to determine the cause. If it's an aneurysm, you may require emergency surgery. For bacterial meningitis, intravenous antibiotics should be given as soon as possible.

MENTAL CHANGES

Watch for confusion, memory lapses or odd or impaired thinking.

Best-case scenario: Mild depression...stress ...low blood sugar...or a deficiency in vitamin B-12.

Worst-case scenario: Severe depression... brain tumor...encephalitis...or an adverse drug reaction. Many drug combinations could cause this reaction, but antihistamines and sedatives are particularly suspect.

Important: Discuss possible drug interactions with your doctor and pharmacist before taking any new medication.

Seek emergency treatment: If disorientation is sudden and acute, mental changes could reflect a serious problem with the central nervous system. Therefore, a prompt evaluation is critical.

See your doctor: With mild or gradual symptoms, get a checkup within 24 hours.

RECTAL BLEEDING

Be concerned if you pass a dark black or maroon stool...or see bright red blood on toilet paper or in the bowl.

Best-case scenario: Hemorrhoids or a tear in the lining of the anus (fissure) can cause bright red blood...iron supplements or Pepto-Bismol can cause black stool.

Worst-case scenario: Rectal cancer when blood is bright red...or colon cancer, bleeding ulcer or diverticulosis (outpouchings, or sacs, usually in the large intestine) if stool is black or maroon.

Seek emergency treatment: If stool is black or maroon and accompanied by dizziness or lightheadedness, you could be suffering from internal bleeding triggered by a stomach ulcer or diverticulosis. Treatment includes blood transfusions and surgery.

See your doctor: For black stool not attributable to iron supplements or Pepto-Bismol, get evaluated as soon as possible. For bright red blood, get a checkup within two weeks. Don't assume hemorrhoids.

UNEXPLAINED WEIGHT LOSS

If you lose your appetite or drop more than 5% of your body weight, despite normal eating, something is wrong.

Best-case scenario: Mild depression...diabetes...overactive thyroid (hyperthyroidism)...or intestinal parasites.

Worst-case scenario: Severe depression...cancer...hepatitis or other liver disease...tuberculosis...or chronic inflammation of the intestinal wall (Crohn's disease).

See your doctor: Get a complete physical, including a thorough blood workup, within two weeks.

VISION DISTURBANCES

Don't shrug it off if you experience blurred or cloudy vision, wavy lines, redness, intense pain or itching in the eye.

Best-case scenario: Allergies...diabetes...pink eye (conjunctivitis)...or outdated corrective lenses.

Worst-case scenario: A retinal tear or detachment...glaucoma...inflammation of the muscular lining of the eye (uveitis)...or foreign matter in the eye.

See your doctor: Have a checkup from an ophthalmologist within 24 hours.

How to Survive a Heart Attack

William Cole, MD, director of the Coronary Care Unit at New York Downtown Hospital, and clinical assistant professor of medicine at New York University Medical Center, both in New York City.

Heart attack kills approximately 500,000 Americans every year, making it the number-one cause of death in the US. But for every fatal heart attack, many more heart attacks do not prove fatal.

Why do some people succumb while others survive? *We can learn important lessons from heart attack survivors...*

DON'T IGNORE SYMPTOMS

When most people envision a heart attack (*myocardial infarction*), they tend to picture someone clutching at the chest, falling to the floor and losing consciousness. This scenario actually describes *cardiac arrest,* when the heart stops beating. The typical heart attack is far less dramatic.

Problem: Heart attack sufferers are often stoic. When they experience chest pain or other symptoms suggestive of heart trouble, they think, *It must be something I ate.*

Why do some people delay seeking treatment? In most cases, the individual was too frightened even to consider the *possibility* of a heart attack…or reluctant to risk embarrassment by calling an ambulance only to find out the problem was heartburn.

These individuals wait hours—often until they're in agony—before seeking help. By the time they reach the emergency room, irreversible damage may have been done.

The most common symptom of heart attack is pain in the chest. But in some cases there is no pain—just a sensation that has been described as "someone sitting on my chest." The pain may radiate up the neck and down the arms.

Other symptoms: Sudden sweating, shortness of breath, tightness in the jaw or nausea.

In some cases, these signs occur several days before an attack. Because the sensations wax and wane, patients are tempted to ignore them. That's a *big* mistake.

Those who are at obvious risk for heart disease—smokers, overweight people and individuals with high blood pressure or elevated cholesterol—should be especially alert to all these signals.

But heart attacks also strike—and kill—people with *no* known risk factors. If you or someone you know notices even mild symptoms, *call a doctor at once.*

GET TO THE HOSPITAL QUICKLY

When treatment is initiated during the first "golden" hour following a heart attack, mortality is only 1% to 5%. After four to five hours of delay, the mortality rate climbs to 12%.

Just 10 to 15 years ago, the death rate associated with heart attack victims who reached the hospital alive was 15% to 20%. Doctors could do little more than administer oxygen and morphine—to make the patient more comfortable.

Now: The death rate for these patients is 5% to 7%. Doctors have "clot-busting" drugs that actually restore blood flow to the heart. But the patient still needs to reach the hospital right away.

Helpful: Call 911 first. Then have someone call your doctor so he/she can alert the hospital

that you're on your way. If the cardiac care team is expecting you, you'll be treated without delay.

GET AGGRESSIVE TREATMENT

Since the early 1980s, heart attack patients have received *thrombolytic therapy*—intravenous drugs that dissolve blood clots. The most effective clot-busters are *tissue plasminogen activator* (tPA) and *streptokinase.*

In addition, nearly all heart attack patients receive aspirin (to thin the blood) and *heparin* (to prevent arteries from re-closing).

While thrombolytic treatment has brought about a significant decline in heart attack mortality, we can do *much* better. Studies suggest that the surgical procedure known as *acute angioplasty* is even more effective than clot-busting drugs.

In this procedure, an X-ray called an *angiogram* is used to pinpoint the blocked coronary artery. Then a small balloon is inserted into the artery through a catheter. The balloon is inflated, pushing aside the blockage and restoring blood flow to the heart.

Problem: Not all hospitals are equipped to perform angioplasty. If you must choose between two hospitals a similar distance away, ask to be taken to the one that is better equipped to do acute angioplasty. If this choice would prolong your trip by 15 minutes or more, it's probably better to go to the closer hospital.

PREPARE FOR EMERGENCIES

If a patient is at high risk of cardiac arrest, it's a good idea for his family members and co-workers to know cardiopulmonary resuscitation (CPR). In fact, *everyone* should learn CPR.

High-risk patients include people who have had prior episodes of cardiac arrest…have a weak heart muscle as a result of a prior heart attack or bypass surgery…or have a history of life-threatening irregularities in the heartbeat (arrhythmias).

These patients might also want to consider asking their doctor about purchasing their own defibrillator. That is the twin-paddled device doctors use to shock the heart into a normal rhythm.

Newer, "smart" models are simple enough to be used by almost anyone—even without training. When placed on the victim's chest, these devices automatically monitor arrhythmias and—if necessary—administer a shock.

Unfortunately, the expense—thousands of dollars—puts personal defibrillators out of the reach of many patients.

Some high-risk patients have been fitted with *implantable* defibrillators. These generally cost thousands of dollars as well.

Stroke Survival

Thomas G. Brott, MD, professor of neurology and director for research at the Mayo Clinic in Jacksonville, Florida. While serving as director of the Stroke Research Center at the University of Cincinnati Medical Center, Dr. Brott helped to develop one of the most successful citywide emergency stroke treatment programs in the US.

Every 45 seconds, an American suffers a stroke. Unfortunately, one in three people does not recognize the symptoms quickly enough to benefit fully from state-of-the-art diagnostic methods and treatments.

If you—or someone you know—suffers a stroke, your response time in seeking medical treatment can mean the difference between full recovery and permanent disability or death.

CAUSES OF STROKE

Think of stroke as a "brain attack." It occurs when the flow of blood—and the oxygen it carries—to the brain is interrupted.

Result: Body functions controlled by oxygen-deprived brain cells may be weakened or lost.

In an *ischemic* stroke, the more common type, a blood clot blocks a blood vessel, usually an artery. This type of stroke is typically painless, but causes weakness, paralysis or loss of sensation on one side of the body…loss of vision in one eye…sudden confusion, trouble speaking or understanding…and/or staggering or inability to walk.

With a *hemorrhagic* stroke, rarer and more dangerous, the blood vessel bursts, leaking blood into the brain or surrounding area. This usually causes a severe headache…difficulty breathing…nausea…and/or vomiting.

Good news: The clot-busting medication known as *tissue plasminogen activator*—or tPA (Activase)—is effective at preventing brain damage, but only in ischemic stroke victims because it promotes bleeding and only if it is administered within three hours of the onset of symptoms.

EVERY MINUTE COUNTS

When you experience or witness even one stroke symptom, call 911 immediately. Stroke victims may be unable to speak to medical personnel, but a family member or friend can help ensure proper care. *Here's how…*

An up-to-date list of all medications the patient takes is crucial for appropriate stroke treatment. Make sure that such a list is in his wallet and/or posted on the refrigerator. That's where emergency medical technicians (EMTs) routinely look for this information.

Next best: Put the patient's medications in a paper bag and take it to the hospital.

When the ambulance arrives, ask the EMTs to take the patient to the nearest hospital that uses tPA.

Remind the EMTs to notify the hospital's emergency room that a possible stroke patient is en route. This allows the ER staff to notify the hospital's stroke team or neurologist on duty… and ask the laboratory to be ready to do blood tests immediately.

DIAGNOSIS

In the ER, the physician should take the patient's vital signs and request a computed tomography (CT) scan or magnetic resonance imaging (MRI) scan to identify what type of stroke has occurred, its precise location in the brain and the extent of the damage.

When tPA is administered intravenously for about one hour or via a catheter directly into the brain, it dissolves 60% to 80% of stroke-related blood clots.

Danger: The drug can cause life-threatening brain hemorrhage if it is used beyond the three-hour cutoff…in patients who have suffered a hemorrhagic stroke…or in people who take the blood thinner *warfarin* (Coumadin).

In patients who are not candidates for tPA, treatment involves controlling the heart rhythm, stabilizing blood pressure and monitoring brain function.

For all stroke patients, the doctor should also order tests that examine blood flow to the brain to determine the cause of the stroke.

Common causes of stroke: Blockage of the blood vessels in the neck or brain from hardening of the arteries...blood clots in the aorta, the artery that leads to the heart...and blockage of the small blood vessels in the brain, often related to high blood pressure.

HOSPITALIZATION

Stroke patients who have suffered a hemorrhagic stroke...received tPA...or are in serious or unstable condition are typically transferred from the ER to the intensive-care unit. Other stroke patients are admitted to a general neurological unit. Doctors then watch for medical complications. Because a stroke can affect breathing, movement and swallowing, pneumonia can develop. A blood clot in a leg vein can move to the lungs, causing a life-threatening pulmonary blood clot (embolus).

REHABILITATION

Within two days of the stroke, rehabilitation typically begins in the hospital's rehab unit. Patients work with physical, speech and occupational therapists to relearn basic skills, such as eating, dressing and walking.

Depending on the severity of the stroke, patients continue their rehabilitation at home or at an inpatient rehabilitation facility. Although some patients do require long-term care in a skilled nursing facility, up to two-thirds of stroke survivors do regain their independence within one year.

Important: Notify a physician if the stroke patient develops a fever of 101°F or higher. This can be a sign of infection or another serious complication.

Up to 30% of all stroke patients develop depression. The signs include persistent sadness... and/or changes in sleep habits or appetite. Such patients should consult a psychiatrist or other experienced psychotherapist.

How to Fight Back If an Insurer Says *No*

Vik Khanna, principal, State Health Policy Solutions, LLC, and author of *Managed Care Made Easy*. People's Medical Society.

Odds are that you will be denied coverage for a health insurance claim at some point in your lifetime.

To challenge the denial, you can file a grievance with the insurance company. But what if the insurer rejects the claim—again? *Don't give up, and here's why...*

Almost all US states offer an external appeals process that allows you to present your case to an independent professional or organization. In about half of these cases, the consumer wins. Effective September 2010, the Affordable Health Care Act has implemented rules to simplify the appeals system for consumers—but the process still varies according to what each state allows. In states where the appeals process is not available, you should consult an attorney on your rights to challenge an insurer's denial of a claim.

To appeal an insurer's decision, such as denial of a surgical procedure or a major diagnostic test, write a letter that briefly describes why you believe the service should be covered. Be sure to include your group number and policy identification number.

Your doctor should also write a letter and provide published research that supports the requested treatment or test.

Because state laws vary, check with your health plan or your state insurance commission—listed under "Government" in the telephone book—to find out the deadlines and rules, including where to mail your appeal.

Send the materials by certified mail. In most cases, you will receive a response within 60 days—and sometimes more quickly if your case is urgent.

To learn more about the appeal rights for Medicare beneficiaries, consult your beneficiary handbook or access the Medicare Rights Center Internet site at *www.medicarerights.org*. You can also get questions answered over the phone—call 800-333-4114.

How to Get Your HMO to Cover Alternative Medical Treatments

Alan Raymond, author of *The HMO Health Care Companion: A Consumer's Guide to Managed-Care Networks.* HarperPerennial.

All HMOs rely on primary care doctors to provide or approve most care for their members. They also tend to cover only "medically necessary" and "nonexperimental" treatments.

Therefore, HMOs might not be willing to reimburse members for alternative medical treatments, such as acupuncture, biofeedback, massage therapy and chiropractic care.

But such treatments are growing in popularity. More than one-third of all Americans have already tried at least one of them.

Here is how to get your HMO to pay for alternative approaches…

• **Find out if the HMO must pay for the treatment in your state,** and under what circumstances. Some states now stipulate that health insurers pay for certain treatments—especially chiropractic care. Your state's insurance department can provide details.

• **Convince your primary care physician to recommend an alternative treatment.** Explain how it will likely succeed in treating your medical problem. Some HMOs will pay for alternative treatments—if you get a referral from your HMO doctor. Call the HMO to find out its policy.

• **Ask your employer to add alternative therapies to your benefits.** Some HMOs do offer riders that expand coverage to include nontraditional therapies. This will cost your employer more, so you will probably receive somewhat higher premiums as a result. The larger the number of your fellow employees who want such a benefit, the more likely it is your request will be granted.

• **If treatment is denied coverage, use tax-sheltered money.** Many employers offer flexible spending accounts (FSAs), which permit you to set aside pretax dollars to pay for uncovered medical expenses.

Acupuncture and chiropractic care qualify, since the IRS has decided that both are tax-deductible medical expenses. The IRS hasn't ruled on other treatments, so check with your employer. Also, find out if you need a medical doctor's referral before getting your treatment.

Medication Errors Can Be Avoided…Easily

Joe Graedon, a coauthor of *The People's Guide to Deadly Drug Interactions* and *The People's Pharmacy: Completely New and Revised.* Both from St. Martin's Press.

Each year, mistakes involving prescription and over-the-counter (OTC) drugs cost the US economy approximately $20 billion in hospitalization expenses…and kill almost 100,000 Americans.

Here's how to avoid "medication misadventures" —taking the wrong drug…overdosing…suffering a drug-induced allergic reaction, etc.

INTERACTING WITH YOUR DOCTOR

Prior to every doctor's appointment, write down in order of importance all your medical concerns and/or symptoms. If you do suspect that a skin rash or any other new symptom is drug-related, make that a priority. This type of problem could be life-threatening.

Most doctors have a limited amount of time to spend with their patients, so it is essential to start with the most urgent problem. If you ramble on about several other problems, the doctor may interrupt you—or you might become sidetracked —before you reach the important one.

Occasionally, the psychological stress caused by seeing a doctor makes it hard to "take in" everything the doctor says. In such cases, take along a tape recorder. That way, you can record the doctor's comments and review them when you're more relaxed.

Important: Be as diplomatic as possible when making your recording. Let the doctor know that you simply want to avoid any confusion following his instructions.

69

Alternative: Ask a friend or family member to accompany you to your appointments. Have him take written notes regarding the doctor's instructions.

NEW PRESCRIPTIONS

Before accepting any new prescription, be sure to provide your physician with the following information...

• **A complete list** of all prescription, OTC and recreational drugs you take, including vitamins, cold remedies, alcohol and tobacco.

• **Any allergy or sensitivity** you may have to any food or drug.

• **Any special diet** that you may be following.

• **Any condition** for which you are already receiving a doctor's care.

Women: Let the doctor know if you are pregnant or attempting to become pregnant.

Ask the doctor for written information about the drug, its side effects and how to take it. If possible, read this literature before you leave the office, but also ask for a copy to take home with you.

Questions to ask: Are there any precautions or warnings of which you should be aware? Should you avoid certain foods, drugs or vitamin supplements while taking the medication?

Failure to get answers to these questions can cause serious problems—even death.

Example: The family of antidepressants called MAO inhibitors (Marplan, Nardil and Parnate) is extremely dangerous when taken in combination with certain other antidepressants...or with OTC cold preparations or diet aids (Acutrim and Dexatrim). Avoid foods with high tyramine content (cheese).

Never take any medication without knowing its purpose. Is the drug intended to alleviate symptoms? If so, which symptoms? Is it intended to cure an ailment? Which ailment?

Obtain explicit instructions about how the medication is to be taken. A simple "three times a day" is inadequate. Find out the correct dosage and at what times of day the drug should be taken.

Ask if the medication should be taken with food or on an empty stomach.

What if you miss a dose? Should you take the dose as soon as you think of it? Or should you simply skip that dose and "double up" on the next one?

Your doctor should double-check for potential interactions between your new prescription and any medications you're already taking. He should not rely on his memory. Instead, he should consult a reference text or a computer program.

If you do experience any unexpected side effects once you begin taking a new medication, let your doctor know right away. Have your doctor tell you which side effects or symptoms require immediate attention.

Caution: Do not stop taking the medication without consulting your doctor. Abruptly stopping certain medications can trigger irregular heart rhythms, convulsions or even heart attack.

AVOIDING PHARMACY MISTAKES

Some patients routinely ask their doctor to "phone in" their prescriptions to a pharmacy. Doing so can be a big mistake—especially when a new prescription is involved.

Reason: Drug names often sound alike—especially when heard over the telephone in a noisy drugstore. The ulcer medication *Zantac,* for instance, can easily be confused with the antianxiety medication *Xanax.*

Your doctor should provide you with a written prescription form. This form needs to be printed clearly, in English, including the drug's brand and generic names, along with detailed instructions. Abbreviations should not be used.

Do not accept sloppy handwriting. In a survey, more than half of pharmacists acknowledged that a doctor's sloppy handwriting had caused them to make prescription errors.

Example: One patient who was supposed to get the anti-inflammatory drug Tolectin was instead given Tolinase, a diabetes drug. She developed *pseudoinsulinoma*, a serious condition that mimics excess insulin production.

Bottom line: If you can't read the prescription, odds are the pharmacist won't be able to either.

To further minimize errors, make sure your prescription is filled by the pharmacist. Because pharmacy technicians have less training than pharmacists, they are more prone to errors. If you are not sure who is filling your prescription, ask.

Finally, visit your pharmacy between the hours of noon and 3 pm. In most drugstores, that's the slowest time of day. Avoid having a prescription filled immediately before or after work. That's the busiest time of day.

DRUG INTERACTION SELF-DEFENSE

Use one pharmacy for all your family's prescriptions. That way, you can be certain that the pharmacist is familiar with all your medications …and alert to potential interactions.

If possible, locate a pharmacy that uses a computerized patient profile system to track the various medications family members are taking. Ask the pharmacist to check the computer for potential interactions. Be prepared to wait—or come back at another time—if the pharmacist needs to check your prescription with your doctor.

Your pharmacist should also check your new prescription for possible interactions with alcohol …or with OTC medications. *Such interactions can cause big problems…*

Example I: The antibiotic tetracycline can be rendered inactive by a single Tums tablet.

Example II: Even small quantities of alcohol can cause a serious reaction in someone taking an antihistamine, tranquilizer, sedative or pain reliever.

Like your doctor, your pharmacist should provide you with instructions on how to take the medication, its potential side effects and any foods or drugs to avoid.

The Eight Most Common Medication Mistakes and How to Avoid Them

Harold Silverman, PharmD, a pharmacist and health-care consultant in Washington, DC. He is author of *The Pill Book: The Illustrated Guide to the Most-Prescribed Drugs in the United States.* Bantam.

Many people unwittingly decrease the effectiveness of the drugs they take—or worse, cause themselves significant harm—by mishandling their pills. *The most common mistakes and how to avoid them…*

MISTAKE #1:
FAILING TO DOUBLE-CHECK YOUR PRESCRIPTION

Drug-dispensing mistakes are rare, but they do occur.

In his haste, a doctor may prescribe the wrong drug or dosage. The pharmacist might misread the doctor's handwriting…or reach for the wrong bottle of pills when filling your prescription.

Self-defense: Before handing the prescription form to the pharmacist, jot the drug name and dosage on a piece of paper.

When you pick up the bottle of pills, compare the label with your note. If you suspect a mistake, call your doctor.

Also, consider keeping a copy of *The Pill Book* (Bantam) or *Physicians' Desk Reference* (Thomson Healthcare) on hand. These books contain photos of pills.

MISTAKE #2:
BEING UNAWARE OF A DRUG'S SIDE EFFECTS

Doctors are supposed to tell patients about a drug's possible side effects. But they don't always do so—because they do not want to "scare" their patients.

Prescription drugs can cause a wide variety of troublesome side effects, including sexual problems like diminished sex drive, impotence and retrograde ejaculation (in which semen is ejaculated "backward" into the bladder). If you are unaware that your medication is causing such a problem, you may worry yourself sick.

Self-defense: Before taking *any* newly prescribed drug, ask your doctor and pharmacist about side effects.

If you experience a problem, ask about taking a lower dose or switching to a substitute.

MISTAKE #3:
TAKING DRUGS THAT MAY INTERACT

Nine out of 10 pharmacies now have sophisticated drug-dispensing software that screens for drug interactions.

Every time you come in with a new prescription, the pharmacist will run a computer check. If the drug does interact with any other drug you're taking, the pharmacist alerts you.

But such systems work only if you have all your prescriptions filled at one pharmacy.

If you patronize different drugstores, you risk subjecting yourself to side effects and/or not receiving the drug's full benefits. You may even fail to discover that you have two prescriptions for the same drug from different doctors—and are double-dosing yourself.

Self-defense: Stick to one pharmacy. If you're taking several drugs and are uncertain about the interactions, ask your pharmacist or doctor for a "brown bag" session. Put all the drugs you take in a bag, and bring it in. Review the name and dosage of each drug, and what each is for.

Be sure to schedule your brown bag session in advance. Otherwise, the pharmacist or physician may be too busy to spend enough time with you.

MISTAKE #4:
COMBINING PRESCRIPTION AND
NONPRESCRIPTION DRUGS

In recent years, several drugs that used to be available only by prescription have gone on sale over-the-counter (OTC).

This cuts costs for consumers, but it makes it harder for doctors to monitor their patients for potentially dangerous drug combinations.

Example I: In rare cases, nonsteroidal anti-inflammatory drugs (NSAIDs), such as *ibuprofen* (Motrin), *naproxen* (Aleve) and *ketoprofen* (Orudis), can cause kidney damage. If you have kidney disease, avoid high doses. Do not take them on a long-term basis.

Example II: The acid blocker *cimetidine* (Tagamet) interacts with the antidiabetes medication *sulfonylurea...benzodiazepine* tranquilizers like Valium...and calcium channel blockers like Adalat and Procardia.

Self-defense: If you're taking a medication on a long-term basis, ask your doctor if any OTC drugs interact with it.

Or—buy your OTC drugs where you have your prescriptions filled, and check with your pharmacist before taking the two together.

MISTAKE #5:
STORING DRUGS INCORRECTLY

No doubt you have already heard that heat and humidity degrade drugs. Yet most of us continue to store our medications in the bathroom—the hottest, most humid room in the house.

Even if you cannot discern any degradation, your pills probably are becoming less potent.

Self-defense: Store all prescription and OTC drugs in a cool, dry spot—your bedroom closet, for example.

If you have children in your house, make sure to keep the drugs out of their reach.

MISTAKE #6:
NOT TAKING THE CORRECT DOSAGE
FOR YOUR WEIGHT

If you lose a lot of weight, a once-correct dose may become a harmful overdose. Conversely, a significant weight gain may lead to under-dosing.

Self-defense: If you lose or gain more than 10% of your body weight, alert your doctor so that he can adjust your dosage accordingly.

MISTAKE #7:
USING PRESCRIPTION DRUGS WITHOUT
MEDICAL SUPERVISION

Many people will hang on to unused pills, thinking they will save a few bucks—and a trip to the pharmacy—if they get sick again.

Yet even if you get the same symptoms again, prescribing to yourself in this fashion is dangerous. Your new symptoms could stem from a different ailment—which calls for different treatment.

Self-defense: If you have pills left over after taking a full course of medication, discard them. If you insist on hanging on to unused pills, at least call the physician and get his approval before using them.

MISTAKE #8:
DISOBEYING YOUR DOCTOR'S ORDERS

When it comes to prescription medications, an amazing number of people simply don't follow their doctor's directions.

Some patients take more medication than was prescribed—on the erroneous "more-is-better" theory. Others take less than the doctor ordered—in a misguided effort to avoid side effects. Physicians call this type of behavior "patient noncompliance."

Self-defense: Take all medications according to instruction. If you have trouble remembering to do this, develop a plan to jog your memory at the appropriate times.

Jot down your dosing schedule in your date book...carry your pill box in your pants pocket as a constant reminder...or pick up a combination pill box/alarm at your local pharmacy.

If you miss a dose, check with your doctor or pharmacist about what to do. In some instances, it's best to continue with your regimen as if you hadn't missed a dose. In others, it's better to "double up" on a subsequent dose.

Avoiding Drug Errors

David W. Freeman, former editorial director, *Bottom Line/Health*, 281 Tresser Blvd., Stamford, CT 06901.

Doctors are notorious for having awful handwriting. Making the problem worse, many common medications have similar names—Accupril and Accutane, Lovastatin and Lotensin, Prilosec and Prozac…to name just a few.

Bad handwriting plus confusing medication names can cause big trouble.

Real-life example: A doctor wrote an order for 2 milligrams (mg) of the blood pressure drug *Cardura* on a patient's hospital chart. But the pharmacist read the doctor's scrawl as 2 mg of the anticoagulant *Coumadin.*

Luckily for this patient, a nurse caught this potentially lethal error and called the doctor, who cleared things up. Of course, not every nurse is as vigilant.

How does one guard against these errors? Diane D. Cousins, RPh, a prescribing-error authority with US Pharmacopeia, the nonprofit organization that sets national drug standards, said that each time a doctor writes a prescription for you, insist that he write legibly. *In addition…*

• **Avoid use of Latin words** and abbreviations for drug names and directions for use.

• **Include a brief notation** of the drug's purpose.

• **Include your age and weight.**

• **Write a zero before a decimal point** (for fractional doses)…but not a zero after a decimal point. For example, 0.5 mg instead of .5 mg, but 3 mg instead of 3.0 mg.

Please take the time to see that your doctor complies. It just might save your life.

Unexpected Side Effects From Common Drugs

Jay S. Cohen, MD, author of *Make Your Medicine Safe: How to Prevent Side Effects from the Drugs You Take* (Avon) and *Over Dose: The Case Against the Drug Companies* (Tarcher/Putnam). *www.medicationsense.com.*

About 40% of the people who take prescription drugs experience side effects …yet many don't make the connection between their symptoms and the medications they are taking.

SUBTLE SYMPTOMS

Antidepressants, such as Paxil and Prozac, may bring on diminished desire for sex. This symptom is frequently mistakenly attributed to stress, lack of sleep or relationship problems.

Zocor and Lipitor, which are taken to lower cholesterol, can bring on many symptoms that mimic the flu. Physicians can easily miss the connection, but muscle aches may signal tissue breakdown. That can lead to serious kidney damage.

Be suspicious of any alterations in your behavior or in the way you feel after beginning a new prescription, especially if the drug you are taking has only recently been approved by the US Food and Drug Administration (FDA).

THE UNCERTAINTY FACTOR

Product information sheets do list common side effects, but that information may not be the whole story…

• **Limited data.** Initial side effects are based on the experiences of people who have taken the drug *before* it was approved for widespread use. Preapproval studies include a relatively small number of people over a limited period of time.

Many drug side effects, therefore, are discovered only after a drug is put on the market.

Additional consideration: The population studied is often not representative of the general public. People who are very sick or who must take several medications, for instance, are often not included in the clinical studies. Women are also frequently underrepresented in drug studies.

• **Unexpected side effects.** These may be serious.

Example: The drug Rezulin, which was approved for use in treating diabetes, was found—before approval—to cause a small amount of liver irritation in some cases. After the drug was in widespread use, however, it caused at least 80 deaths and hundreds of cases of severe liver damage before it was taken off the market.

• **Unique response.** Drug companies anticipate certain side effects based upon reactions of the sample population. But—every individual is a special case. So your experience may not be the same as that of another person.

DOSAGE DANGERS

As many as 80% of side effects are dosage-related. If you begin taking a new drug, ask your doctor if it is possible to start with a lower dosage. For many people, a lower dosage is just as effective as a higher one...and with minimal side effects.

Better Than Viagra?

Men who burned approximately 200 calories daily through physical activity—the equivalent of a brisk two-mile walk—were less likely than sedentary men to become impotent, one study has found.

Moderate daily exercise delays the normal, age-related slowdown in the production of testosterone, which is necessary for erections.

Good daily exercise: Walking, jogging or swimming.

Caution: Men who bicycle for more than three hours per week have a higher risk for erectile dysfunction.

Irwin Goldstein, MD, editor in chief, *The Journal of Sexual Medicine*, Boston.

Glucosamine Alert

Although it's generally quite safe, research suggests that glucosamine increases insulin resistance in both diabetes sufferers and those at risk for the disease. An early sign of type

2 diabetes, insulin resistance—a decrease in the body's response to the hormone insulin—promotes unstable blood sugar levels.

Self-defense: Diabetics and people at risk for diabetes should monitor their blood sugar levels carefully when using glucosamine...and ask a doctor whether the supplement may be increasing their risk of diabetes or making the disease worse.

Chris Foley, MD, board-certified internist, Minnesota Natural Medicine, St. Paul.

Folic Acid Danger

The synthetic forms of folic acid can trigger hives, breathing problems, cramps as well as itching.

Problem: The US Food and Drug Administration (FDA) is urging food producers to fortify bread, flour and pasta with folic acid...and many vitamin supplements now contain folic acid.

Self-defense: Consult a doctor if you develop these symptoms after a meal—or while taking vitamins containing folic acid. (Also, stop taking the vitamins.)

Good news: You can get plenty of natural folic acid by eating dark-green leafy vegetables, liver, nuts and wheat germ.

Mark Dykewicz, MD, director and professor, pulmonary, critical care, allergy and immunologic medicine, Wake Forest University Baptist Medical Center, Winston-Salem, North Carolina.

Calcium Supplements Are Not Created Equal

Avoid the calcium supplements made from bone meal or the mineral *dolomite*. These supplements are sometimes laced with arsenic and lead. Generally, low lead levels in calcium supplements are unlikely to be a health risk because calcium blocks lead absorption. People over the age of 65 often have a deficiency of digestive acid and should take calcium with food or juice or use a *calcium citrate* supplement, which requires less stomach acid for absorption.

Barbara Levine, PhD, RD, associate clinical professor of nutrition in medicine, Weill Cornell Medical College in New York City.

Green Tea Warning

Green tea, which has become popular for its anticancer effects, can interfere with the action of the prescription anticoagulant *warfarin* (Coumadin).

Recent case: A 44-year-old man was taking warfarin to prevent postsurgical blood clots. The drug's effectiveness declined unexpectedly, raising the man's risk for potentially deadly clots. When they investigated, experts discovered that the man had been drinking up to one gallon of green tea a day. When he gave up the tea, the effectiveness of the drug was restored.

Theory: Green tea contains vitamin K, which interferes with the anticoagulant effect of warfarin.

Green tea and vitamin K–containing foods, such as spinach and cabbage, are safe to consume in moderation.

James R. Taylor, PharmD, clinical associate professor of pharmacy practice at the University of Florida College of Pharmacy, Gainesville.

The Value of Herbal Ingredients

Do not pay extra for vitamin supplements with herbal ingredients. Herbal substances are of questionable value, and may interfere with vitamins in a manner that blocks your body from absorbing them. So you may wind up paying more for less.

David B. Roll, PhD, director, dietary supplements, United States Pharmacopeia (USP).

Sodium/Cataracts Link

A high amount of sodium in your diet can lead to cataracts. Adults consuming the most sodium were twice as likely to develop *posterior subcapsular cataracts*—a type of cataract that covers the back of the eye lens—as those consuming the least.

Self-defense: Limit sodium intake to between 1,500–2,400 milligrams a day.

Robert G. Cumming, MPH, PhD, professor of epidemiology and geriatric medicine, University of Sydney, Australia. His two-year study of 2,873 adults was published in the *American Journal of Epidemiology*.

Cold-Water Warning

If you have coronary artery disease, uncontrolled high blood pressure or a disorder of the peripheral vascular system, such as Raynaud's syndrome, it is not safe to do a cold-water plunge at a spa or health club. Sudden exposure to the cold-water temperatures could cause your arteries to spasm, which can lead to stroke.

How it works: A cold shower or plunge will stimulate the autonomic nervous system, which controls heartbeat, blood pressure and other involuntary functions. Blood pressure and heart rate temporarily spike when you're exposed to cold, but return to normal levels after the plunge. If you have mildly elevated blood pressure (not above 140/90), it should decrease to healthier levels with regular cold-water treatments.

Start by immersing or spraying your feet, hands and face with cold water. Wait at least a week before taking a full-body plunge—and limit it to 40 seconds. If you still feel cold 10 minutes later, you overdid it. Always precede a cold-water plunge with a hot shower or bath.

Alexa Fleckenstein, MD, a Boston–based practitioner of traditional and complementary medicine.

75

Sunscreen Alert

When shopping for sunscreen, search for the products that contain the ingredient *avobenzone* (Parsol 1789). This substance protects against long-wave ultraviolet (UVA) radiation. The majority of sunscreens protect only against short-wave radiation.

Good brands: PreSun Ultra and Ombrelle.

Robert Bissonnette, MD, founder and president of Innovaderm Research and MedQualis, clinical research firms located in Montreal, Canada. Dr. Bissonnette's study was published in *Archives of Dermatology*.

Basil Repels Mosquitoes

Rubbing a handful of fresh basil leaves on your skin should protect you from mosquitoes for a few hours. The herb does not contain hazardous chemicals and is less likely than synthetic bug sprays to cause skin irritation. It's also cheaper.

James A. Duke, PhD, a Fulton, MD–located author of numerous books, including *The Green Pharmacy* (St. Martin's), and former chief of the US Department of Agriculture's medicinal plant laboratory.

Be Your Own Personal Trainer and Save $45 an Hour

Miriam E. Nelson, PhD, an associate professor and director of the John Hancock Center for Physical Activity and Nutrition at Tufts University in Boston. She is also coauthor of the *Strong Women* series of books and the founder of *www.strongwomen.com*.

If you exercise regularly, then you probably already know the value of a good personal trainer.

A trainer can help you to establish and maintain a regular exercise schedule...recommend appropriate workouts...push you harder for better results...and teach you proper form and technique. But trainers typically charge $45 or more* for a one-hour session.

Good news: It's possible to get results on your own—without a trainer. *Here's how...*

A REGULAR SCHEDULE

• **Work out with a friend.** Commit to specific times and days each week. You are less likely to miss a workout if another person is counting on you.

• **Make a realistic time commitment.** How much time can you devote to exercise each week? Thirty minutes per day? Thirty minutes three times a week? If you set unrealistic goals, you're likely to quit.

Choose the days you'll exercise, then write them in your calendar. Check them off once you've completed each workout.

Helpful: Think of each exercise session as an "appointment" with yourself.

Having difficulty fitting your routine into a busy schedule? Try exercising before work or during your lunch hour...getting up early two mornings per week...dropping a low-priority item from your schedule...or performing three 10-minute workouts, rather than doing one 30-minute session.

• **Choose a suitable location.** Look for a convenient site that provides the services and equipment you need.

If winters are severe where you live, exercise indoors. Buy a stationary bicycle or treadmill, or use an exercise video.

When traveling, stay at a hotel with a fitness center. Ask the concierge for a walking or running route. Or pack a jump rope.

• **Keep a detailed exercise log.** Charting your progress over time will motivate you to maintain your program.

Include the date you exercised...how long you worked out...and the specific routine you performed.

Note at the bottom of the log the intensity of each routine—*too easy, just right, too hard*. This helps you recognize when a routine is no longer challenging.

Example: February 15...40 minutes...running and weights...intensity—just right.

*All prices subject to change.

For a weight-training routine, list the type of exercise…pounds or level of the workout…and number of repetitions.

THE BEST ROUTINES

There are three basic types of workouts…

• **Aerobic exercise.** Brisk walking, jogging or bicycling increases the heart rate.

• **Strength training.** Lifting weights preserves muscle strength and function.

• **Flexibility training.** Stretching expands your joints' range of motion.

Find a routine that satisfies your requirements for exercise, such as preventing back pain or tightening your abdomen.

Participate in aerobic exercise at least three times a week…strength or flexibility training at least twice a week. Begin each session with five minutes of easy exercise, warming up to full intensity. Finish up with a five-minute cool down that includes stretching.

THE RIGHT INTENSITY

Exercise won't do you much good unless you work out at an appropriate level of intensity.

To "push yourself" just as a personal trainer would, ask yourself after your workout…*Could I have exercised longer? Could I have done more difficult exercises?* If so, increase your intensity next time.

Or you might be exercising too hard. Ask yourself after the routine…*Am I exhausted? Do my limbs feel heavy and sore?* If so, decrease your intensity.

Exercise physiologists have devised these exercise intensity guidelines…

• **Aerobic activity.** At least three times a week for a minimum of 20 minutes, exercise at a level that requires strenuous movement, elevating your heart rate to 60% of its maximum.* Breathing is rapid. Sweating starts within 15 minutes.

Incorporate into your daily life easy, sustainable movement that increases your heart and breathing rates slightly.

Sample activities: Strolling…gardening…golf.

*To measure heart rate: Locate your pulse on your neck or wrist. Count the number of beats for 15 seconds and then multiply by four. *To calculate maximum heart rate:* Subtract your age from 220. If you're age 50, for example, your maximum heart rate is 170.

Avoid overexertion. You have overdone it if your heart is pounding to the point of discomfort or nausea, or if breathing becomes too rapid for you to speak easily.

• **Strength training.** During the first four weeks—while you are learning the exercises—work out at a moderate exertion level. This causes fatigue only if prolonged, like carrying a full bag that gets heavier as the day goes on.

Stabilize at a level that begins at moderate intensity and gets harder after six or seven repetitions. You should be able to maintain good form while performing the movement eight times, but you will need to rest afterward.

Avoid any movements that require all your strength. These can cause injuries to bones and muscles.

• **Flexibility training.** Hold the pose and push it to the maximum stretch—but not to the point of pain. And *never* bounce.

Smart Ways to Do Medical Research

Carol Svec, a Raleigh, NC–based researcher, medical writer and patient advocate. She is the author of *After Any Diagnosis: How to Take Action Against Your Illness Using the Best and Most Current Medical Information Available.* Three Rivers Press.

I f you have always trusted your doctors to stay up to date on medical treatments, you are taking a big chance.

Every year, more than 3,000 biomedical journals are published. Every year, the US Food and Drug Administration (FDA) approves more than 500 new or updated drugs and more than 3,000 new medical devices. No doctor can keep up with all these innovations.

Patients must fill in the gaps by becoming experts on any medical condition from which they suffer. Studies do indicate that informed patients spend fewer days in the hospital, lose fewer days of work, feel less depressed and report lower levels of pain.

EASIER SEARCHES

The Internet has made gathering medical information easier than ever before. There are thousands of Web sites where you can learn about specific diseases and conditions.

To find reliable information, start with Web sites that are sponsored by government agencies (with URL addresses that end in *.gov*), educational institutions (*.edu*) or nonprofit organizations (*.org*).

Find one or two good Web sites and consult them periodically. For common disorders, such as diabetes, multiple sclerosis or asthma, checking back once a month is sufficient. For rare diseases, once every six months is plenty, because breakthroughs occur so infrequently.

Exception: For life-threatening diseases, check *every week* for updates and information on new clinical trials.

Do not let the search become an obsession. Gathering information may help you feel "in control," but when the paper chase starts controlling you, it's time to scale back the search.

USING INFORMATION WISELY

Some physicians do not reveal all medical options to their patients—because they think patients will be confused by the choices or because the doctors specialize in a particular treatment.

Example: A surgical oncologist may be more inclined to recommend treating cancer with surgery, rather than with radiation or chemotherapy.

If you're well-informed, you will be able to discuss all the treatment options, make sound medical decisions and avoid health scams.

Work in partnership with your physician. Doctors know medical facts, but patients know how they feel. *Good ways to stay involved...*

•**Talk openly with your doctor** about wanting to participate in your own care. Most physicians encourage their patients to become active information seekers. If your doctor objects, find a new one.

•**Keep your physician in the loop.** Don't try any new medication, supplement, herb or device without discussing it with your physician. Make sure it won't interfere with your current treatment.

•**Stay in touch *between* doctor visits.** Questions often arise between office visits. Ask your doctor how he prefers to respond to these inquiries.

Good choices: Sending e-mail (if you are not worried about privacy), talking on the phone after office hours or consulting a nurse or physician's

assistant. If these strategies do not work, you might have to book a separate appointment.

•**Don't deluge your doctor with written material.** Bring no more than three articles to your physician per visit. That's all he will be able to evaluate during a typical appointment.

•**Track your progress.** Request copies of all your medical reports (blood tests, X-rays, etc.) and keep them in a file. Log all monitoring information, such as blood pressure or glucose levels. Note any changes since your last office visit, including new pain or other symptoms and steps you've taken to control them.

Bring your file to each doctor's appointment. This information lets the doctor know what's happening between office visits, and it provides a quick reference in case you change doctors or require emergency care.

STOP SCARING YOURSELF

Health statistics can be confusing and frightening. When assessing these numbers, remember that they are based on the *average* outcome of research involving thousands of patients.

Example: If a disease is said to have a 50% death rate, the statistic is based on reports from a broad sample of people who have had the disease. This includes those who had extensive treatment and others who opted for no treatment.

Statistics are utilized for understanding the seriousness of a disease, but statistics should never be used to predict an individual's outcome. Numbers alone should not make you lose hope. *Before you worry over a study reported in the news, find out...*

•**Did the study involve humans?** Animal studies are a valuable first step, but the same results are not always found in people.

•**How many people participated in the study?** The more, the better. If a study uses fewer than 100 subjects, don't take its results too seriously.

•**Were the participants similar to you?** Did they have the same disease? Were they of the same sex and of a similar age? Unless the subjects were people just like you, the study may not be relevant.